CW00503995

OUR GUIDE TO UNDERSTANDING PREMATURE OVARIAN INSUFFICIENCY

Daisy Network

Grosvenor House
Publishing Limited

This book is published by
Grosvenor House Publishing Ltd
Link House
140 The Broadway, Tolworth, Surrey, KT6 7HT.
www.grosvenorhousepublishing.co.uk

A CIP record for this book
is available from the British Library

ISBN 978-1-83975-741-9

Foreword

If you're here reading this book, the chances are you've been diagnosed with premature ovarian insufficiency (POI), are suffering some of the symptoms and haven't yet got a diagnosis, or you're reading it in support of a loved one who is dealing with the condition. Whatever your reason for finding us, we welcome you and hope that you find a little bit of comfort from being as informed as possible and knowing that you're not alone.

Daisy Network was founded in 1995 by a group of patients under Dr Gerry Conway who were either themselves suffering from POI or were the mothers of daughters with the condition. In the early days it started as a support group run by women in their spare time, giving them a chance to meet up with others in the same situation over a coffee and a chat. Today we have expanded into being a registered international charity, but Daisy Network continues to be run totally by volunteers.

As someone who was diagnosed with POI at the age of 16 years, I would like to start by saying that I understand what you're going through. Each volunteer at Daisy Network each has their own reason for supporting the charity and whether they have gone through POI themselves, have a family member with the condition, or are a medical professional who works with women with POI, they are all passionate about the cause.

Daisy Network is the only registered charity supporting women with POI and, although we are based in the UK, we have branches and volunteers offering support across the globe.

POI can be a lonely diagnosis as it's still a relatively unknown condition and our aims are to raise awareness of the condition and provide a safe space for women to find support, not only from medics but from each other. We also aim to provide more knowledge to the medical community, as currently there are many women not getting the necessary support from their healthcare professionals, purely due to the condition not being a priority in medical training.

One thing I get asked a lot in my role as chair of Daisy Network, is 'are there any books on POI I can read?' The simple answer is No. Although there are plenty of useful resources available on aspects of POI and menopause, there is no up-to-date book which focuses specifically on POI as a condition.

So to follow the Daisy ethos of spreading the word about the condition and because we are approaching the 25th anniversary of Daisy Network, we as a team, are collating our knowledge and experience together to bring you this guide to POI.

Amy Bennie – chair of Daisy Network

With huge thanks to our wonderful Daisy Network team of volunteers who generously donate their time and knowledge to the cause, without whom the charity wouldn't be able to function. And to our incredible and courageous Daisy Network members, who have so kindly contributed their personal POI stories in order to help others.

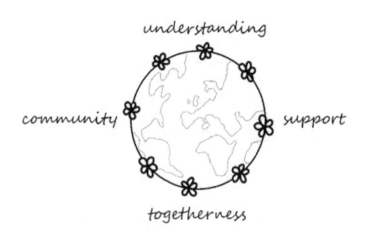

understanding

community

support

togetherness

Chapter 1

What is POI?

So you've probably been told that you've got one of three things, premature ovarian insufficiency (POI), premature ovarian failure (POF) or premature menopause. Let's be honest, whichever term was used, none are particularly great.

I know a lot of women have googled 'POF' and the first search result is the dating site *Plenty of Fish*, not exactly what you want to see when you've just been given a difficult diagnosis.

The problem with the terminology is that it doesn't really explain what the condition actually is. Have your ovaries failed? Are they deficient in something? The word 'premature' also comes with its own negative connotations. The term 'premature menopause' is probably the easiest to understand, most of us know about the menopause, even if just through thinking of your gran having a hot flush and blaming it on 'the change'. Menopause is simply the name given to the last menstrual period. As your periods tend to stop with POI this term does make sense as you've prematurely stopped having periods. But it doesn't quite explain the condition in full. For example, a teenager whose ovaries have not yet begun to function, or someone whose ovaries have been surgically removed, are suffering POI and don't have periods but it's not because the menopause came early. No wonder it can be so confusing to understand what it is that you've been diagnosed with.

While there is no internationally agreed wording, the preferred term for the condition is premature ovarian insufficiency (POI), which may describe it more accurately as POI differs from the menopause in many ways and in some cases, the ovaries may still ovulate occasionally and have therefore not irreversibly 'failed'.

The European Society of Human Reproduction and Embryology (ESHRE) guidelines define POI as: 'a clinical syndrome defined by loss of ovarian activity before the age of 40 years characterised by menstrual disturbance (amenorrhea or oligomenorrhea) with raised gonadotrophins and low estradiol.'

In layman's terms it means that the ovaries aren't working as they should (*why couldn't they just say that?*). They stop producing eggs years and in some cases even decades before they'd 'normally' be expected to. In addition, the ovaries are unable to produce the required amount of hormones oestrogen and progesterone, which have important roles in women's health and well-being. It is the low hormone levels, particularly oestrogen, that cause many of the symptoms associated with POI such as hot flushes, night sweats, vaginal dryness and mood disturbance. Additionally, oestrogen is very important for long-term bone, heart and brain health.

We will be referring to the condition with the official terminology, POI, in this book but whether you call it premature ovarian insufficiency, premature ovarian failure, or premature menopause, it's important for you to take control of your diagnosis and use the term you feel most comfortable with and the one that resonates with your personal experience.

'When I was diagnosed with the condition, I really hated that it was called early menopause. I felt too young, I didn't have symptoms and it didn't feel like it fit with what I was going through. The term POI works much better with how I feel and what I have experienced.'

Jenny

POI Affects:

1 in 100 women under 40
1 in 1000 under 30
1 in 10000 under 20

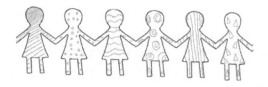

(We must also mention, just to cause more confusion, that if your ovaries stop working under the age of 45 but after the age of 40 it's defined as early menopause, not POI.)

As the reason for the ovaries not working varies from person to person, nearly everyone with POI has a different experience. Some find their ovaries stop working before they even start their periods, for some it comes out of nowhere after having a seemingly regular cycle, whereas others might be prepared and informed that they will go through POI after surgery.

We are born with all the eggs contained in our ovaries that we will ever have, usually around one to two million. The number of eggs in our ovaries, also called ovarian reserve, usually declines gradually with age so that just a few thousand are left at menopause. If you're born with a lower egg number, or the egg count reduces more quickly, then you may develop POI.

There are five main reasons why your ovarian reserve might reduce prematurely and lead to POI. These are:

1. Idiopathic – in around 90% of women of all ages with POI, the condition happens spontaneously with no known cause or reason for it. The shock and lack of preparation for this huge life change, as well as not knowing why it happened to you, can be really tricky to deal with.

2. Auto-immune – around 5% of women are thought to have developed POI as a result of an auto-immune disorder where the body's immune system attacks its own tissue mistaking it for a threat. If this happens, the ovaries can become damaged resulting in POI. Some specific auto-immune conditions which are known to be linked with POI are Hashimoto's Disease, Type-1 diabetes and Addison's disease. If you get diagnosed with any of these conditions, it's worth mentioning POI to your specialist.

3. Genetics – abnormalities in the female sex chromosome (the X chromosome) or other genes affecting sex hormone function can cause POI. The most common genetic defect of these is Turner syndrome, where one of the X chromosomes is missing. POI is also associated with some rare conditions which tend to run in families such as Fragile X syndrome and Galactosaemia.

4. Infection – there have been reports of POI occurring after infections such as mumps, tuberculosis and malaria but these occurrences are extremely rare.

5. Surgery/Treatment – surgical removal of the ovaries before the age of 40 years is another cause of POI. This sudden removal of the site of hormone

production can often lead to an abrupt onset of the menopause. Removal of the ovaries (with or without hysterectomy) can be required for several reasons including ovarian cancer, ovarian cysts, endometriosis or severe premenstrual syndrome. Hopefully, this type of surgery will be planned in advance, so you would have the opportunity to discuss with your specialist what might happen. As well as surgery, other cancer treatments such as chemotherapy or radiotherapy can cause temporary or permanent damage to the ovaries, resulting in POI. The chances of this occurring depend on the chemotherapy drugs used, the site of radiotherapy and your age at the time of treatment.

Although most women will not be given a clear reason as to why they developed POI, the majority of cases are likely related to genetics. Approximately 10–15% of women with POI will have a mother or sister who also has it. People often worry that their POI was caused by something they did, like taking the contraceptive pill or having too much stress, but for most women it's caused by things completely out of your control - mainly your genes.

In Summary

POI happens when a woman's ovaries stop working, before the usual age of menopause. It can happen naturally, or as a side effect of some treatments. Because the ovaries are no longer functioning, or have been removed, they don't usually ovulate or produce the hormones oestrogen, progesterone and testosterone.

The Best View Comes
After the Hardest
Climb

Chapter 2

Signs and Symptoms

As with a lot of POI related things, it isn't a straight forward process. There are no specific set of symptoms that can be used to confirm that you are suffering from POI, but the most common reason women feel there might be something wrong is due to noticing a problem with their periods.

Teenagers might find that they never actually start their periods and are late going through puberty, which could be a sign of POI. The National Institute for Health and Care Excellence (NICE) guidelines suggest that not starting your periods by the age of 15 years, or periods which stop for six months after they started, could indicate that you need to get checked for POI.

A lot of women with POI notice that their periods become erratic or stop completely. I bet you're all thinking *'this has happened plenty of times to me'* and there lies the problem. Periods becoming irregular can happen for so many reasons. It is usually recommended that you see your doctor if your periods have become irregular over three to four months or longer. Another common factor is that so many women take some form of hormonal contraception which overrides the action of their own ovaries. Unbeknown to them, their ovaries may have stopped working long before they even realised. It's often the unfortunate situation where women spend so much of their life trying to avoid pregnancy that it's only at the point where they are actively trying to get pregnant, they realise there is a problem.

Aside from changes to periods, the sudden drop in oestrogen when the ovaries stop working can cause a plethora of symptoms that usually make women feel rubbish enough that it warrants a trip to the doctor. So how do you know when your oestrogen level has dropped? This is where the menopause side of POI comes into play as you might start experiencing those nasty menopausal symptoms. Here is a list of the typical symptoms women may get. Some women may unfortunately suffer with all of them, some only one or two.

SYMPTOMS

Physical

Irregular or no periods
Hot Flushes and Night Sweats
Palpatations
Weight Gain
Skin and Hair changes
Headaches
Breast Tenderness
Joint or muscle Pain
Vaginal Dryness
Infertility
Urinary tract infections

Psychological

Insomnia
Mood Swings
Irritability
Anxiety
Panic attacks
Loss of self esteem
Lowered Libido
Difficulty concentrating
Memory lapses
Low energy levels
Depression

By speaking to women with POI you realise how differently it affects each individual. Some suffer badly with the physical symptoms: sweats, insomnia, headaches, whereas others suffer mentally, with symptoms like anxiety, mood swings and depression.

'I thought I was going crazy, my brain didn't seem to function, I was waking up in the night drowning with sweat and my moods were all over the place. I'm not usually an emotional person but I just felt so up and down it wasn't like me. This went on for about a year, I just kept thinking it will pass, or it might be stress or being overworked. At 32 menopause didn't cross my mind but it was talking to my mum who had similar symptoms when she went through early menopause, that made me push to get blood tests.'

Abbie

Most often when girls are diagnosed as teenagers, they don't tend to get these menopausal symptoms. As the ovaries stopped working so early, oestrogen levels haven't actually built up to their full peak yet, so the hormonal drop, which is what causes the symptoms, isn't as drastic.

With such a variety of symptoms, it's easy to see why a diagnosis can be tricky. The difficulty is that many of these are common complaints and can be attributed to life events, stress, hormone fluctuations or just feeling under the weather. Who hasn't experienced one or more of these symptoms at some time or another? This can lead to frustrating delays in diagnosis as many women tend to wait a while to see if the symptoms will pass and it's only after months or years of feeling rubbish, that they decide it's probably time to go to the doctor.

Alone we are strong.

Together we are stronger

Chapter 3

Getting a Diagnosis

A passion of ours here at Daisy Network is to raise the awareness of POI with doctors. When a young, healthy woman comes into a clinic with irregular periods, whilst most commonly it isn't something to worry about, it often takes a while for POI to even be considered as a possibility. The training on it is very minimal and it often depends on each individual practitioner as to whether they have much knowledge about the condition.

Postcode lottery is something we hear a lot when it comes to fertility and women's health and this also applies to POI. Some doctors will look after their patient's POI care themselves, referring them for scans and handling medication and tests. Other doctors will refer the patient to a specialist, whether it's an endocrinologist, gynaecologist or menopause clinic. There is not a set route to go down with POI diagnosis and treatment and it's unfortunate that your level of care depends on who you're seen by. Our aim is for everyone diagnosed with POI to be referred straight away to a specialised clinic to get the best care by people who truly understand the specifics of the condition. POI is sometimes just treated the same way as 'normal' age menopause but there is so much more to it that shouldn't be missed and so much more training is needed for the condition to be fully understood.

The NICE guidelines recommend a referral to a specialist for holistic management of POI: 'Consider referring women with premature ovarian insufficiency to healthcare professionals who have the relevant experience to help them manage all aspects of physical and psychosocial health related to their condition'.

* * *

So you have arrived at the doctors, explained your symptoms and the doctor suggests some tests. What will happen next?

Blood tests

If your doctor follows the NICE guidelines, the first port of call will be getting a blood test to measure your levels of follicle stimulating hormone (FSH). This is the hormone that the brain releases to tell the ovaries to release an egg. FSH levels above 30iu/L (international units per litre of blood) are an indicator that the ovaries are failing and menopause is approaching or has happened. The brain uses FSH to tell the ovaries to ovulate. With POI, the ovaries have stopped responding so the brain releases higher and higher amounts of FSH to try and shout at the ovaries to work. If your FSH levels are high this indicates that the ovaries aren't responding.

If you're still having periods, it's really important that the FSH test is done between days two and five of your cycle, otherwise the results may not be accurate. If your periods have stopped completely then it doesn't matter when the blood test is done. Your doctor may also do some other blood tests at the same time to look for other causes of irregular or absent periods including testosterone and prolactin levels and thyroid function tests.

If you are under the age of 40 and have had two blood measurements of high FSH taken four weeks apart, in combination with absent or irregular periods, this provides a diagnosis of POI. Measuring the oestrogen level at the same time can help to confirm a POI diagnosis. If the ovaries aren't functioning, they won't be producing oestrogen, meaning that the levels in the blood will be low.

Your health professional might then choose to follow up with some additional tests to see if there is anything else going on that may be the cause. These tests can include genetic testing and testing for autoimmune disorders, depending on your age and medical history.

FSH levels can fluctuate widely, particularly in the early stages of POI. This variation can sometimes make the diagnosis more difficult. If there is any doubt your doctor should refer you to a menopause or reproductive medicine specialist.

Scans

Depending on your healthcare professional, you might get sent for a set of scans. The first is a pelvic ultrasound.

This can help to see if there is anything physically wrong with the ovaries or uterus which may be causing irregular or absent periods, such as polycystic ovarian syndrome. The ultrasound can also help to see how many follicles are remaining in the ovaries, as sometimes if the diagnosis is caught early enough, there may be a chance to do some fertility treatment. It's quite common with teen girls to find their ovaries and uterus are small and underdeveloped if POI has happened before puberty has finished.

Oestrogen is a major factor in keeping bones strong and healthy, so a dual energy x-ray absorptiometry (DEXA) scan is useful to see if low oestrogen through POI has had any impact on your bones. A DEXA scan is a kind of x-ray that scans different parts of the body, usually the hip bone and legs and measures the density of your bones. Low bone density can cause osteoporosis, a condition which means your bones are brittle and can break very easily. Usually this can be managed with hormone replacement therapy and supplements such as vitamin D and calcium but it's better to have this checked sooner rather than later before it gets too severe.

You may not control all
the events that happen to
you, but you can decide not
to be reduced by them. -
Maya Angelou

Chapter 4

Treatment

Treatments for conditions are sometimes thought of as cures, and while there is currently no way to reverse or get rid of POI, treatment is vitally important to maintain wellbeing and manage the condition. In general oestrogen therapy is the main treatment option recommended both for the management of symptoms of oestrogen deficiency and its long-term effects. The most common treatments are hormone replacement therapy (HRT) or the combined oral contraceptive (COC) pill.

Hormone replacement therapy

If you've been diagnosed with POI, taking HRT is recommended until you reach the age of natural menopause, which is considered to be 52 years old in the UK, although you can continue to take HRT for a longer period of time if you want, there is no limit. Similar to menopause, even the term HRT comes with a whole host of stigma and is something you will have heard people talking about and possibly in a negative way. I know personally when my specialist told me it was time to change from the pill to HRT, it really hit me and made me realise, *wow, I really am in the menopause*. It's something so regularly associated with older women, it can feel aging for young girls, I remember my specialist telling me not to worry, that lots of young girls take HRT, it's not just for old ladies. I have to admit, it didn't help.

I'm sure you will all be familiar with the scare around HRT and breast cancer that was widely publicised in the 1990s. But please rest assured that taking HRT when you're under the natural age of menopause does not carry these (albeit minute) risks. Think of it like this; if women each have a tall glass, those without POI would have a glass full of water (oestrogen) and those with POI would have a glass that was nearly empty. Those with POI are taking HRT to fill up the empty glass to the same level as others their age. As we are lacking oestrogen and only increasing it to the correct level we need to function, there is no risk of breast cancer.

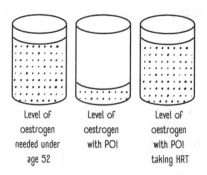

Level of oestrogen needed under age 52

Level of oestrogen with POI

Level of oestrogen with POI taking HRT

There are very few women with POI who can't take HRT. Women who are considered high risk for HRT (mainly those with hormone-sensitive cancers such as breast cancer or endometrial (uterine) cancer) should be referred to a specialist to discuss their treatment options.

It's important that doctors take an individualised approach to HRT as everyone's background is different and there is no 'one size fits all' method HRT.

The hormones used in HRT are:

- **Oestrogen** – the hormone responsible for relieving symptoms experienced and also used for the protection of the skeletal system, cardiovascular system and brain function. It may originate from plant sources. It is different from the oestrogen found in the contraceptive pill, which is of synthetic origin and is more powerful than natural oestrogen.
- **Progestogens** – given alongside oestrogens if you still have your uterus. There are many varieties of progestogens but all have the same role which is to protect the uterus lining from becoming thickened from stimulation with oestrogen.

There are three main types of HRT:

- **Oestrogen only HRT**
  For women who have had their ovaries and uterus removed by a hysterectomy. Because the role of progesterone is simply to protect the uterus, this group of women do not need progesterone and are therefore usually prescribed oestrogen only HRT.
- **Cyclical HRT**
  Contains oestrogen and a progestogen and will produce regular bleeding. Also sometimes referred to as sequential HRT. Used for women who still have irregular periods or prefer to have a monthly bleed and usually only for the first couple of years after diagnosis.

- **Continuous combined HRT**
  Contains similar hormones to cyclical HRT (oestrogen and a progestogen) and is used for women who do not want to experience a bleed or have been bleed free for two years or more.

Some women choose to take HRT that doesn't produce a period, however if you're hoping to either conceive naturally or have fertility treatments such as IVF egg donation, it's usually recommended to have a withdrawal bleed to keep the uterus lining healthy.

* * *

Tablets

HRT comes in many varieties and it can be a case of trial and error to find the form that best suits your body and your lifestyle.

Oestrogen

Tablets are the most commonly prescribed form of oestrogen. They're easy to take and the dosage given is simple to adjust should you need to. Through the skin methods, such as gels, patches and sprays, present an advantage as they go directly to the bloodstream, whereas tablets have to be metabolised by the liver. Again it's completely down to the individual which they feel best taking. HRT patches, gels or sprays are more appropriate for women with a history of blood clots, high blood pressure or migraines.

Progesterone

If you still have your uterus, the oestrogen needs be used along with a progestogen to keep the uterus lining healthy. There are lots of different ways of taking progesterone. It sometimes comes combined with oestrogen in tables and patches. It also comes separately in tablets, vaginal gels and hormone containing intrauterine systems (the hormonal coil).

Bioidentical hormones

There has been a lot of interest recently in the concept of 'bioidentical hormones' as HRT. Bioidentical hormones mean exact duplicates of the hormones produced by the ovaries – oestrogen, progesterone and testosterone. These can be prescribed on the NHS and are commonly used in women with POI however we don't have enough evidence to say whether they are better than those used in non-bioidentical HRT.

It's important that these bioidentical hormones aren't confused with compounded natural hormones – often called 'bioidentical' as a marketing tool. These are produced by compounding pharmacies and are often delivered by cream or lozenge. These products are not licensed or regulated and therefore there is no data to show whether they are safe or effective. For all menopausal women, and particularly those with POI, we don't recommend compounded hormone treatments like these as we just don't know whether they are safe and protect your health in the long-term.

TYPES OF HRT

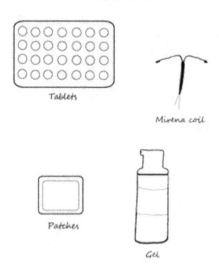

Tablets

Mirena coil

Patches

Gel

Testosterone

Testosterone gel is also part of HRT you might want to consider. This can be the missing piece of the puzzle. Testosterone is often thought of as a male hormone but women also produce the hormone and it has a really important role throughout the body and it has a really important role throughout the body. Oestrogen hormone replacement helps menopausal symptoms to stop and protects long term heart and bone health, but a lot of women find that taking additional testosterone alongside, gives them the extra boost of energy they are lacking and improves libido. Taking testosterone can be a necessity for some, especially those women who have POI due to surgery and no longer have ovaries. Androgens may also have important positive effects on mood, wellbeing, energy and vitality in women.

Testosterone is available in the form of a gel or cream. Testosterone gel is currently only licensed for use in men in the UK and would be used in a smaller dose for women only under specialist advice. At the moment it's usual to offer testosterone therapy only to women who are already using oestrogen treatment. Don't worry, the aim of treatment is to bring women back to their necessary physiological range and provided these dosages are followed, you should not experience side effects such as increased facial hair or deepening voice.

Vaginal Oestrogen

One of the common symptoms of POI is vaginal dryness. Taking systemic oestrogen in the form of a tablet, patch or gel, can sometimes help vaginal symptoms but often extra oestrogen is needed. There are vaginal tablets, gels, creams or rings which can be used in addition to your other HRT that are very effective. This is a local treatment which doesn't go into the blood stream so is very safe. A year's worth of vaginal tablets provides the same dose as taking as one single oral tablet. We do suggest if you're suffering bad vaginal symptoms to always check with your doctor.

Combined Oral Contraceptive Pill

If you find that HRT doesn't suit you, the combined oral contraceptive (COC) pill is an alternative option. An advantage of the contraceptive pill is that it's widely used, easily available, and as most women take it anyway, it can provide a sense of normalcy for those with POI. An added bonus of COC is that as it's a contraceptive, you don't have to pay a prescription charge, whereas often with HRT containing double hormones it can come with a double charge. (At Daisy Network we are currently working alongside the Prescription Charge Coalition to try and change this).

Both the COC and HRT can be good at managing the symptoms of POI but we still don't know if they are equally effective at protecting against the long-term effects of oestrogen deficiency on the heart, bones and brain. The NICE guidelines and a paper by Langrish et al, 2017, both show that HRT may be slightly more beneficial for bone and heart health than the contraceptive pill but there aren't enough long-term studies on this subject to know for sure.

If you're trying to decide between HRT and the COC it's also worth bearing in mind that HRT isn't a contraceptive (except when using the Levonorgestrel Intrauterine System – the hormonal coil). As some women with POI may have spontaneous ovulation, if pregnancy isn't something you would want, the COC can be a good option.

Getting the right treatment can be the key to feeling yourself again.

HRT Troubleshooting

As we mentioned previously, HRT isn't a 'one size fits all' form of treatment and even if you do have one that suits you, you might still get some side effects.

Oestrogen side effects

Mild side effects from oestrogen can be quite common when you start HRT. These 'start-up' effects include breast tenderness, nausea and headaches. They are usually mild and settle after a few weeks, so we usually suggest trying to persevere for two to three months before changing or stopping treatment. If these side effects carry on for longer, or are more severe, changing to a transdermal oestrogen (patch, gel or spray) rather than a tablet may help, or reducing the dose and building it up slowly.

Progestogen side effects

The body produces progesterone which is one of a family of progestogen molecules. There are a wide range of different progestogens used in COC and HRT. Progestogens can have premenstrual syndrome (PMS) type side effects including mood changes, bloating, acne, breast tenderness and headaches. For women suffering these side effects there are several options. Generally taking micronised progesterone (instead of one of the other progestogens) is associated with fewer side effects. Also using a progestogen-secreting intrauterine device (coil) often suits people better as the hormone works directly on the uterus lining and less is absorbed into the bloodstream.

Irregular bleeding

Irregular bleeding or spotting is quite common in the first four to six months after starting continuous combined HRT. If it continues for longer than this, or you start bleeding after a long time without periods, then you should see your doctor. Sometimes you need a pelvic ultrasound to ensure there is no thickening of the uterus lining or polyps. Your doctor may recommend changing the type, dose or route of progesterone to help with the irregular bleeding.

The advantage with HRT is that there are so many different forms and methods of taking it and it can be tailored to suit your needs. It is important that you find something that fits in with your lifestyle and doesn't give you side effects. It can take a while to find the right form and dose for you but it's worth persevering to find something you're happy with. Furthermore, if your doctor is struggling to find a method of HRT that suits you, they should refer you to a specialist menopause/POI clinic.

Vaginal Dryness

Glands around the neck of the uterus and at the entrance to the vagina, produce natural lubrication to keep the vagina moist and clean and to aid sexual intercourse. The low levels of oestrogen in POI cause changes to the vulva and vagina causing them to become thinner, drier and less elastic (known as vaginal atrophy). This can cause pain, particularly during sex, which can have a knock on effect on your libido, or when inserting tampons, but in some women even a light touch from clothing can be painful. Other symptoms of vaginal dryness include itching, burning, changes to your vaginal discharge and difficulty having smears. It's not uncommon for people to think they have thrush or an STI. It can also affect the tube from your bladder (urethra) making you want to go to the toilet frequently. These symptoms can really affect your quality of life but it's often difficult to talk about them or get your health professional to take them seriously but it's worth persevering as there are lots of effective treatments.

- Local oestrogen. As discussed previously vaginal oestrogen is very effective at treating vaginal dryness and comes as a range of different products which can be used in addition to your usual HRT
- Local DHEA. This is an androgen-like form of testosterone. Vaginal DHEA pessaries taken each night are licensed for treatment of vulvo-vaginal dryness.
- Lubricants for intercourse. There are many different types of lubricant out there which can be applied just before intercourse. Water-soluble or silicone products are usually advised if you're new to lubricants, as oil-based products can sometimes cause irritation. Oil-based lubricants tend to last longer but aren't compatible with condoms. Silicone lubricants aren't compatible with silicone sex toys.
- Vaginal moisturisers. These can be prescribed or bought over the counter and should be used regularly for maximum benefit. They can be used even if you're also using vaginal oestrogen.
- Several lifestyle measures can be really helpful for relieving symptoms as well including avoiding perfumed soaps, tight clothing, douching or using harsh chemicals such as perfumed detergents and feminine hygiene sprays.

She was powerful,
not because she wasn't scared
but because she went on so
strongly,
despite the fear."

— Atticus Poetry

Chapter 5

Fertility

One of the most unfortunate, and often distressing consequences of POI is infertility. While the physical and mental symptoms caused by POI can often be treated through HRT, the lack of ovulation leading to infertility, sadly, can't easily be managed.

The term premature ovarian insufficiency was changed from premature ovarian failure because in some women, the ovaries don't completely fail. Ovarian function can fluctuate over time, occasionally resulting in a period, ovulation or even pregnancy, several years after diagnosis. Due to this intermittent return of ovarian function, approximately 5– 10% of women with POI may still conceive, although this is a rare and extraordinary occurrence.

Unfortunately, for women with POI the usual fertility treatments, such as ovulation induction or invitro fertilisation (IVF), are very unlikely to be successful. In order for these treatments to work, medication is used to stimulate the ovaries to produce eggs. In women with POI as there are very few eggs left, the ovaries do not respond well to these medications meaning that the chances of success are usually less than 5%. It also means that egg freezing isn't usually possible if you've already been diagnosed with POI; this is only usually done for people who are at high risk for POI (such as those undergoing cancer treatment).

If carrying a baby and giving birth is something that is important for you to experience, and you still have a functioning uterus with withdrawal bleeds on your HRT, then pregnancy is possible by using egg donation. IVF using donor eggs is the most commonly suggested and most successful fertility route recommended.

Egg Donation

The use of donor eggs can be a strange concept to grasp. A great analogy compares a donor egg to a box. You are given the flat packed gift box but you're the builder, you put it together and fill it up. Without your effort and materials it would just be a flat packed piece of cardboard, it wouldn't be a complete present. It's the same with donor eggs. While you may not have produced the egg and it has been generously given to you by another woman, by carrying that pregnancy, you shape that baby's genetics for the rest of its life. It's your body and blood that protects and feeds the baby. Without your body, the baby wouldn't exist.

One other route for egg donation which some women may find more comfortable, is the use of a known egg donor. A known donor is pretty self-explanatory, it's someone you know and have chosen to donate their egg, whether it be a relative or sometimes even a friend. This route means you don't have to go on a waiting list to

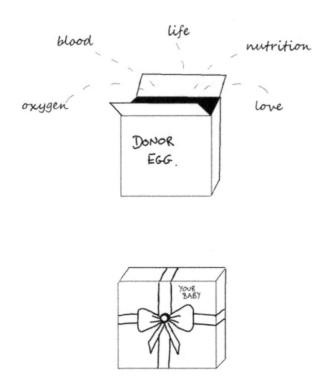

find a donor and you can be have full confidence with who the egg came from, which for some women can bring a huge comfort with who the egg came from. For others, the idea of personally knowing the egg donor, can be uncomfortable. When the child grows up they will usually be around their donor if it's a family or friend and for some this is difficult especially if there is a physical resemblance. The anonymity of an unknown donor can provide distance. However, for a lot of women using a relative as an egg donor, such as a sister, provides that desired genetic connection to their baby. They know they will share the same DNA as their child and the family resemblance will be there. There is also the bonus that with a known donor, often age restrictions are waivered.

They say the time is never right to have a baby, there is always a job, a holiday or a life event that gets in the way of you thinking it's the right time to take the plunge. This is even more-so the case with fertility treatment, it needs planning and preparation and can be a long process which takes a physical, mental and financial toll. The donor conception network is a great resource to support you through the egg donation process.

Adoption

For some women, they just want to be a mother and the pregnancy, baby and genetics aren't important. Adoption is an incredible way to get the family you long for while also giving a great life to a child who needs it. There are currently thousands of children up for adoption in the UK, most of which are siblings and the number of those who actually get placed in an adoption are dropping each year. There is a history of adoption carrying a lot of stigma towards potential parents, yes the process can take a long time and feel invasive but there isn't the judgment there used to be and it doesn't matter whether you're single, married, divorced, LGBTQ+ or have a disability. If adopting a child is something you would like to do, your local authority will have an adoption agency who can guide you through the process.

Positively child free

It's important to remember that POI isn't just about the loss of fertility and for some women this isn't their main concern. Many choose to live positively childfree (you can read Nia's inspiring story further on in the book). Some women embrace the fact they cannot have children and choose to find purpose in life through another form, whether it be their job, travel, animals or their relationships with family and friends. Sometimes the focus after a diagnosis of POI is to figure out the way to overcome infertility but it's important to remember who you were before the diagnosis and what you truly want out of your life.

'After my POI diagnosis, I straight away started to look at my options for getting pregnant. It sort of felt like it was the way to fix the problem. But I looked at the different routes and none of them felt right for me and my partner. I took a while to realise that actually, if I hadn't had POI, I probably wouldn't have even considered having children. My life is fulfilled with my partner and my pets, I'm so happy and realise that I don't need to find a way to have a child to fill a void, because the void isn't there. What I have is all I need.'

Alice

There are some new medical advances going on which may mean one day women with POI can have their own biological children. There have been reports of pregnancies after injection of platelet rich plasma into the ovaries (often known as ovarian rejuvenation) and there are several studies ongoing investigating the therapeutic effect of stem cells in women with POI. Although these techniques are still experimental, this fills us with great hope that the next generation of women with POI may have more options and can be in control of their fertility.

You never know
who you are inspiring

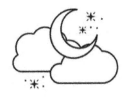

Chapter 6

Psychological Aspects of POI

Because POI is a physical change that happens to you, a lot of medical intervention is focussed on making you feel physically better, replacing those missing hormones, strengthening bones and getting the right levels of HRT to stop the hot flushes and mood swings. Of course this is super important, but POI has a much broader impact than just on our ovaries. POI isn't just a diagnosis affecting the body, it also affects our mind and the psychological impacts aren't always addressed with as much detail and importance.

For most, getting diagnosed with POI will come as a massive shock and it's a life altering thing to be told. We find that depending on the woman's age at diagnosis, the psychological impact is different. Generally when teenagers get diagnosed, it's often the case that the POI diagnosis doesn't sink in straight away. It's usual that they are at a point in life where they are consumed with personal life, school, exams, friends, relationships; not only that but fertility seems a long way away. It's common for teenagers to shut off from the diagnosis until they are older, but there is always the psychological impact of feeling different from peers, and conversations about periods and puberty can cause this to come to the surface. For women who are at the stage in life where they are actively trying to conceive and are ready to start a family, finding out they have POI can be utterly devastating. Even women who already have children or have completed their families, will still feels the psychological affects of POI, such a big life change can feel like an ending that has come too soon with the choice being taken away. Others however, after feeling so unwell, may be pleased to finally have a reason for the way they are feeling.

Puberty, periods, fertility, oestrogen, ovaries, pregnancy are all words we associate with womanhood. A diagnosis of POI can feel like your femininity and identity has been stripped away from you. It's normal to feel like your body has let you down and it can have a huge impact on your self-esteem and body confidence. Those parts of your body that were once associated with womanliness or sexuality, now feel like they are failing and are under scrutiny by the medical profession. Teenagers can especially feel this if POI has halted puberty. Changes like breast development don't happen until a later age which can bring up questions about gender and delay getting into relationships due to embarrassment.

Some women feel a disconnect with sex. The thing that is done to procreate, no longer has that purpose. While, yes, sex is also an enjoyable experience, some women feel like they no longer 'work' so find the enjoyment has been replaced by shame. Medical exams and discussion of your fertility can be an embarrassing thing for most women and the association with those parts of the body and feeling attractive, can change. Similarly, there is still a horrible stigma around the term menopause and it's association with ageing and being less desirable, which can make women with POI feel old before their time.

The fact that women don't physically change on the outside, so POI is commonly a hidden diagnosis, brings with it its own psychological impacts. Yes it means many women still feel confident in their looks but it also means that from the outside others do not understand what you're going through and it can often come as a shock to disclose what you're going through to people, as outwardly, they wouldn't know. It means that women are subjected to unhelpful comments by peers as they assume because you look fit, healthy and attractive, it isn't a topic they need to be sensitive about.

There is also the worry of telling partners. Women tend to worry at what point should they tell their partners when they are in a new relationship. Too early might be too serious too soon, too late may feel like a betrayal. Equally, there can be guilt that having POI is also changing the life plans and hopes of their partner, knowing that having children may be a difficulty or no longer a possibility. What we always say here at Daisy is that most partners are with you for who you are as a human being, not for your fertility and if they don't take it well, then they're not the right person for you.

'Finding out my girlfriend had POI didn't have a negative or detrimental impact on our future together at all, I don't think of her any differently than I did

before. Yes, we may have to consider some different options to have children one day but nothing else has changed. I love her for who she is and if you also have the right person in your life, they will love you for who you are, having a medical condition doesn't change that.'

Loui

* * *

'At least you don't have periods anymore' is a common and insensitive thing that young women tend to hear from their friends, which shows a huge lack of understanding. There's no denying periods aren't pleasant for a lot of people, they are a hassle and can be very painful, but I'm sure if you asked the majority of girls with POI, they would wish they had natural periods.

Your relationships with those around you, can feel like they change after a POI diagnosis. Friends and siblings may feel like they are moving ahead of you in terms of milestones. A shocking diagnosis tends to halt your plans, whether it be relationships, careers, it's usually the case that women feel like they fall behind others. It's also common to feel a sense of isolation when friends or family discuss menstruation.

'I remembered my friend asking me to lend a pad, so I went into my mum's room, got one out her drawer and pretended I'd got it from my own room so she wouldn't know I hadn't started my periods.'

Emily

With teenagers, parents' reactions can have a huge impact on how they deal with the diagnosis. We often see parents wanting to make the teen feel normal, by saying 'everything will be ok' and not discussing the diagnosis by putting it to one side. Unfortunately as they get older, women may feel like the diagnosis was discounted and they have not actually dealt with the true feelings which then come out at a later age. It's important to tread carefully with teens as it's a sensitive and often embarrassing topic but make sure that you're aware how tough it's for them, that it isn't something to be ashamed of or kept secret and that you're open to talk should they want to.

A diagnosis twenties and thirties can be difficult as this is a time siblings and peers may be starting their families. There may be conflict between feeling happy for them but sadness for what you can't have. POI is a loss and a bereavement. It feels like a loss of femininity, a loss of feeling well and loss of your life plan. Having the choice of having biological children taken away from you, should be treated like a bereavement. You're grieving for what you can no longer have, or for the future children you had assumed you would have. We need to go through this mourning process in order to heal.

Counselling or talking therapy can be a really useful tool to help you to process your POI diagnosis. Working through it with a counsellor can help you come to terms with, accept, and understand the diagnosis, and move your life forward in the direction you want.

***

It's extremely important for us to mention, that cultural differences need to be considered during the POI diagnosis, both psychologically and medically. Information has been gathered from personal experiences from our team and members.

Now for the embarrassing part, although it really shouldn't be. Something that is still taboo and not often talked about is the impact POI can have on the mental and physical aspects of sex.

Finding out you can't get pregnant via the 'normal' heterosexual method e.g. man and woman have sex and the woman gets pregnant, can have a huge effect on how women view sex. It often goes one of two ways. The first with the thought, 'excellent, now I can have all the sex I want with zero chance of pregnancy' quite a sexual liberation to come out of an upsetting diagnosis, as so many women spend a lot of their lives avoiding pregnancy. (We would also like to note that there is still the risk of STI's, so barrier contraception is important). But for many, it goes the opposite way, sex become something that is stigmatised with 'not working'. The low self-esteem can make women feel unattractive and sex becomes something with a medical focus rather than for enjoyment. Despite the fact that prior to a POI diagnosis, the aim of the majority of sex isn't to get pregnant, it can become a focus of 'what's the point?' if the outcome of sex will never be pregnancy.

'After my diagnosis, the idea of sex was just a reminder that I couldn't get pregnant. I lost all interest in it, I was worried it would be uncomfortable but I somehow

felt less feminine and ashamed of my own body. I had been prodded and poked so much getting tests that it felt medical, not enjoyable.'

Jen

It's extremely important to note that it isn't just women in heterosexual relationships who feel this way and no matter what your sexual orientation is, your openness to intimacy and sexual stimulation can be compromised. There are sex counsellors out there that can help you work with you on the relationship between your body, sex and POI. Being open in communication with your partner is also key, let them know you may need to take extra time to feel comfortable.

Lots of women with POI become disconnected with the idea of having sex. If the ovaries aren't working, does that mean the other bits won't work properly too? For some women low oestrogen caused by POI can make sex, or any type of stimulation, very painful and they struggle massively with vaginal dryness or atrophy. It's suggested that you use a vaginal moisturiser to ease symptoms, along with a lubricant, we recommend the brands 'Yes', 'Replens' or 'Sylk'. Vaginal oestrogen pessaries, creams or rings can be used in addition to your usual HRT and can be extremely helpful for vaginal dryness.

In some cultures, women's health is something thought of as a private matter, so going through POI can add loneliness as there isn't the ability to confide in those around you. It can come with a shame due to having a family being a top priority.

The acceptance and allowance of fertility treatment is also something that can vary. The use of a donor egg or third party medical intervention in some cultures may not be allowed, which can mean women in these situations have less options or have to go about seeking treatment privately without family knowledge.

There are also certain traditions that are carried out at weddings. For example, only women that have children can take part in a dance routine or seating plans that are created depending on your parental status. For an event that brings people together things can become unintentionally uncomfortable for someone with POI.

(You can read the story written by Anonymous Daisy member further on in the book.)

Chapter 7

Long-term Health

The long term impact on the body from having low oestrogen associated with POI, is something that can be prevented with the correct course of treatment. Using HRT should help to reduce the risk of these conditions by restoring oestrogen to their 'normal levels' but there are still some lifestyle measures which are important to consider.

Osteoporosis

Oestrogen is really important for bone health and without it bone turnover (the total volume of bone that is both resorbed and formed over a period of time), can become abnormal resulting in thin, weakened bones which are at risk of breaking or fracturing. In the early stages this is often called osteopenia and as it becomes more severe it's called osteoporosis. Osteopenia and osteoporosis are usually diagnosed on DEXA scans which are commonly done when you're diagnosed with POI, particularly if there are other risk factors for osteoporosis such as family history, previous fractures, smoking, steroid use or very low body mass index.

For most women with POI diagnosed with low bone density, HRT will be the mainstay of treatment. If you can't take HRT, or your bone density has got much worse while on HRT, there are other treatments that can be used such as bisphosphonates. However, these have certain disadvantages and are usually only used in women with POI under specialist guidance. One of the concerns about bisphosphonates in women with POI is that we don't know about their safety in pregnancy and so they should really be avoided in women hoping to conceive.

It is usually recommended to repeat the DEXA bone density scan after three to five years, although the frequency of this will depend on your baseline result, whether you're using HRT, your background risk factors and local practice guidelines.

Lifestyle and diet can be really important to reduce your risk of osteoporosis. Taking regular weight-bearing exercise will help maintain bone strength. National Health Service (NHS) guidance recommends taking a 10mcg vitamin D supplement daily and ensure your diet is rich in calcium and vitamin D. (See chapter 8 on nutrition, for more information).

Cardiovascular disease and brain health

No long-term studies have yet been conducted in women with POI to look at whether taking HRT reduces our risk of heart disease and cognitive impairment. Short-term studies, however, have shown that HRT has a beneficial effect on the cardiovascular system. HRT is therefore recommended up until at least the average age of menopause (52 years old) in women with POI to help protect the heart and brain.

Not every day is good, but there is something good in every day.

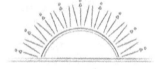

Chapter 8

Nutrition and Wellness – Catherine O'Keefe

www.wellnesswarrior.ie

Food as fuel: the key

Diet is one of the cornerstones of menopause management; what we put into our bodies directly affects our moods, emotions and physical symptoms. You can follow a good exercise routine, practice mindfulness daily but the benefits will be lost if nutrition is not part of your plan. A proper balanced diet will enhance your energy levels and help to address anxiety from a stronger place.

'We are what we eat' – it's as simple as that. Everything we put into our bodies affects our brain chemistry and therefore our energy and our moods. A diet with high levels of sugar and processed foods will cause mood swings, energy spikes and crashes, weight gain, sluggishness. Anxiety, stress, tension, tiredness can all be alleviated by a good, balanced diet.

Take the time to write down what you're eating over one week and it will help you fully understand your habits and pinpoint where you need to improve.

When looking at nutrition, it's very helpful to understand the importance of the neurotransmitters in our bodies and the interaction with the adrenal gland and the pituitary gland. Think of your body as a racing car and your food as the fuel – without the right high-grade fuel your body cannot expect optimum healthy performance. The fuel interacts with all parts of your body with the most important part being the brain, which acts like a centralised computer. The brain sends messages to different parts of the body as and when required through chemical messengers called neurotransmitters.

When anxiety occurs these neurotransmitters send messages to the adrenal gland (secretes adrenaline which acts in the short-term and cortisol which acts over a longer period) and the pituitary gland to raise the fight or flight signal. This results in an increase in energy and blood sugar levels to deal with the threat or perceived threat. Therefore when we look at our diet we must ensure we are supporting and strengthening these key components.

Nutrition Top Ten

1. Watch your blood sugar levels – a steady blood sugar level results in a more balanced mood. When your blood sugar level falls below the normal it causes stress hormones to be released, these are used by the body to release glucose stores which give us energy. While this is useful in a 'fight or flight' situation, an excess of stress hormones (cortisol and adrenaline) only serves to increase

anxiety. So not skipping meals, especially breakfast, is essential to avoid low blood sugar levels.

2. Eat breakfast like a king. It is a good habit if you can include foods that are high in protein or complex carbohydrates, slow release sugars, as these will give you energy until snack time. Breakfast sets you up for the day ahead. Before eating breakfast, adding a sliced lemon to warm water with some fresh turmeric or ginger gives your digestive system a warm fuzzy feeling first thing in the morning. Cinnamon is lovely added to porridge or buckwheat in the morning and is good for blood sugar balance. There is also research now suggesting that cinnamon can enhance brainpower and lead to improved concentration.

3. Eat regular small meals, ideally every three hours.

4. Ensure good sources of fat, protein and carbohydrate are included in all meals, as these will make you feel satisfied, reduce cravings and give you slow-releasing energy.

5. Eat healthy snacks throughout the day – for example sliced apple with almond butter, a boiled egg, hummus and carrots, rye cracker and mashed bananas with almond butter (or any other type of nut or seed spread). You can also find many recipes for protein balls that also make fantastic daytime snacks.

6. Include fresh vegetables and fruit. Eat as much as you can of green leafy vegetables like kale, spinach and broccoli and fresh fruit especially blackberries, raspberries and blueberries.

7. Incorporate sources of Omega 3 into your daily diet. Omega 3 is discussed in more detail later.

8. Eat wholegrain food and avoid processed foods–heavily processed white bread, pasta and rice are quickly broken down into sugars in the body which causing your blood glucose to increase. This rapid increase is often followed by a crash which is evident by cravings or headaches.

9. Avoid sweet treats. Instead go for nuts and seeds as they will keep you fuller for longer, help avoid low blood sugar and provide a great nutrient hit containing magnesium, selenium, B vitamins, calcium and Omega 3. Make or buy nut butters, sprinkle nuts and seeds on salads, porridge etc. If you're really craving chocolate, opt for the dark kind, 80% cocoa solids or up.

10. Take time to enjoy your meals, this can be a great time to practice daily mindfulness. This is easily achieved by sitting down for your meals and eating more slowly, being mindful of each mouthful and consciously enjoying the food you're eating.

A flourishing gut is a flourishing mind

'Gut flora is the housekeeper of the digestive system.'
Gut and Psychology Syndrome

Good gut health

Plenty of research has been done on the gut-brain connection and it's now generally accepted that the two are directly linked, with the gut now being referred to as 'the second brain'. We now know that the gut is responsible for producing a large amount of the body's neurotransmitters, those vital messengers (chemicals) that send information from the brain to the body and vice versa. The stomach is also our first line of defence against illness, providing a barrier to ward off viruses and bacteria with 80–85% of our immunity located in the gut wall (Source: Gut and Psychology Syndrome, 2018).

It is currently estimated that the gut is responsible for 90% of your body's serotonin production – so it's worth looking after! Research also indicates that gut bacteria enhance the production of gamma-amino butyric acid (GABA), which is another essential neurotransmitter that calms the brain.

Probiotics are good bacteria for the stomach and prebiotics are bacteria which act as food for the growth of the probiotics. Both types of bacteria help digestion by keeping the gut clean and everything flowing smoothly. The more prebiotics in your gut the healthier your probiotics, your gut and immune system will be. Prebiotics naturally exist in many foods we consume on a daily basis and as fibre is a source of prebiotics foods high in fibre are usually high in prebiotics.

Use probiotics, prebiotics or fermented foods to encourage a healthy gut bacterium.

- Prebiotic foods include Jerusalem artichoke, garlic, onions, avocado, leeks and bananas. In the raw state the prebiotic content is higher but reduces when cooked.
- Probiotic foods include natural yogurt, kombucha, kefir and fermented foods. Daily intake of milk

kefir morning and evening is a great addition to the diet.

Hydration

Ensure you drink enough water; dehydration is one of the most common symptoms in menopause and can also make your general symptoms worse. So drink extra water, aim for a minimum of six to eight glasses per day (1.5–2L). Take a moment for a cup of herbal tea, slow it down for a few minutes to stop and enjoy the fluid. Any of the following can be a great addition:

- turmeric
- chamomile
- peppermint
- jasmine
- lemon balm
- hot water & lemon
- fresh ginger in hot water
- green tea
- sage (great for hot flushes)
- valerian (particularly at night time).

Foods to limit include:

- Caffeine which is a stimulant and like all stimulants is can increase anxiety, make you more irritable and affect your sleep. Remember too it's also a diuretic, which will only worsen the symptoms of dehydration, which are so common in menopause. Ideally you should eliminate caffeine from your diet slowly, so as not to give your body a shock withdrawal.

- Sugar, alcohol & dairy.
- Processed foods.
- Spicy foods especially if you're also having hot flushes.

Managing Stress

Practice mindfulness

'Don't just do something, sit there.'

Ruby Wax

Mindfulness is well researched for its benefits to our wellbeing and can be used as a way to train your brain to patiently observe your anxiety. Think of it as you would a parent observing a toddler's temper tantrum – you can observe and watch the behavior but need to remain calm and passive until the tantrum is over.

Daily routines can be used as opportunities to practice mindfulness, to focus on the present, on what is happening right now. For mindfulness to become part of your life it must work for you, it must be something you benefit from and not something you dread. In that respect, start small, let it find ways into your life and it will work for you. When sitting in traffic, just be for a few moments right where you are, not on the way to somewhere, or the way from somewhere, not late, not early. Just there, in that moment.

When we stop and sit in 'the now' we can slow down what we are experiencing and take time to savour and enjoy what life has to offer. Being mindful lets our minds be present and become clearer. The realisation that this very moment is all there is and that everything else is merely a thought, projected into the future or excavated from the past is the start of letting go of worry.

Stress fades away and our minds become calmer. It's all about taking life in smaller bites, not hour-by-hour but minute-by-minute. Just focus on the next 60 seconds, and then the next, minute by minute.

Stop constantly doing and simply STOP.

Practical everyday mindfulness

Begin with simple ways to be present:

- Concentrate on the process of making tea – slow down and pay attention to the movement of your hands, the smell of the tea, the steam from the kettle, the sound of the water pouring and finally, the taste of the tea.
- Washing your hands – pay attention to the water, the smell of the soap, the slipperiness of the lather, the movement and sensation of your fingers and palms. Pay attention to only these things for a few moments – this is a meditation of sorts.
- Eating – notice the textures, the colours and the aroma of your food as well as the taste, slow down the action of eating and focus on the sensation of the food on your palate.
- Do a digital detox for one hour during the day.

Meditation

Living in the now – understanding and changing your approach.

Like many meditation novices, I took a long time to develop the habit and to see the benefits. But when I persevered, I realised that the same principle applied to meditation for the mind as exercise for the physical body: repetition and practice increase strength. You don't need to be sitting cross-legged like the famous yogis; you can meditate anywhere (within reason!) that works for you. The benefits of meditation are widely celebrated and once you find what works for you it's a great addition to your daily habits.

Start small. Five minutes per day is enough to get you started and you can use apps (Headspace is excellent), follow CDs, YouTube channels and guided meditations. Find what suits you best.

Sleep

None of us function at our optimum when we have missed a few hours of good deep sleep. Sleep in my view is a fundamental human need, we need sleep to allow our bodies to recharge and for our nervous system to unwind. Sleep gives our body that vital downtime after the stresses of the day. So when you've had a night of hot flushes or night sweats, you will automatically feel more anxious the following day, as your body is tired and therefore more vulnerable to anxious thinking.

Review your sleep hygiene and consider these small tweaks to your nocturnal routine:

- Use the breathing techniques outlined earlier to help you drift off to sleep.
- If you're experiencing night sweats, have a tepid shower before bedtime and have some lemon water bedside.
- Practice good sleep hygiene:
    - A no-tech bedroom – this is crucial for undisrupted sleep. Revert to a battery alarm clock.
    - Establish a social media curfew from 9:00pm every evening.
    - Keep the room as dark and at a comfortable temperature.
    - Exercise during the day, avoid last thing at night.
    - Keep a regular bedtime and awake time to stabilise your circadian rhythm.
    - Declutter your bedroom. Take the time to do this – it will immediately lead to a calmer mind.
    - Avoid caffeine and alcohol in the late afternoon and evening.
- Magnesium powder is also excellent for the nervous system and disturbed sleep patterns.

Self-care

Self-care has never been top of my agenda but I have learned the wisdom of looking after oneself before one can effectively help others. Laughter and smiles are contagious but so too are anxiety and stress. Setting yourself up to be calm and happy for the day ahead will positively impact your family, your work and anyone you meet.

Taking care of yourself is inextricably linked to keeping anxiety at bay. The process of caring for yourself sends a very important message to your brain that you're valuable and that you're safe. Do not be dissuaded by any notions that self-care is selfish. Think of it instead as essential maintenance of the machine we inhabit. We need time out for ourselves, from our relationships, from social media, from family – time out allows us to be a better, calmer, less anxious person and this enables us to engage better with our families and friends.

Think of self-care as nourishment for your head, your heart and your body. When we have energy reserves restored by practicing self-care, we are well equipped to deal with anxiety and stress. Most of the tips outlined in this book can also come under the umbrella of self-care. Create your own personal self-care toolkit to help you navigate your life, to protect you from burnout, to handle hormonal fluctuations and of course, to deal with anxiety.

Self-care is not selfish; it's essential and offers a protective shield against the trails of life and helps you be the best version of yourself that you can be. Think of Mount Etna... you want to avoid a volcanic eruption and small regular self-care habits (pressure releases) will prevent this happening.

Please review the following questions and answer them (honestly) to help provide an outline of how you can be nicer to yourself:

- What makes me smile?
- What do I enjoy doing and could do more of?
- What could I do less of?
- What would I do differently if I knew I was precious and loved myself?
- How would I look after myself?

Use these questions to create a list of your favourite self-care ideas – we are all unique in what we enjoy so dream big on this one.

Indulging in the things that bring you joy is the difference between truly living your life and going through the motions. I know when I am doing anything from my list, I am distracted from negative thoughts, I become totally immersed in what I'm doing because I love and enjoy it so much, there is no time for anxiety or worries to seep in. Try to get a list of at least ten favourite things and then plan to incorporate them into your week.

Self-care and self-esteem

When you experience ongoing anxiety it affects your self-confidence and self-esteem. While positive affirmations might help you feel momentarily better, it's my opinion that anxious people need much more. What is effective is self-care. When you practice daily self-care, you're caring for yourself and engaging with the world around you in a more meaningful way, all of which makes you feel good about yourself, which in turn positively impacts self-esteem. Participation in activities, hobbies that have value to you, taking the time out to do things you enjoy; these simple steps will enhance self-esteem.

I would also include within self-care, avoiding toxic people and negative situations, especially if you're going through an anxious period. Take care of yourself first and when you're in a stronger, calmer place, you can assertively handle the problems.

Exercise

Exercise, like nutrition, is one of the cornerstones of a healthy life. The benefits of exercise are well documented and range from enhanced cardiovascular health and improved sleep to optimal brain health and endorphin release (the natural anti-depressants). Exercise also burns off the stress hormone adrenaline.

This powerful antidote encourages the release of the feel-good chemicals (endorphins) that are imperative in balancing mood swings and reducing stress. The very nature of exercise helps every aspect of health, from building immunity to reducing everyday stress. While you're exercising you're breathing more deeply, your mind is taken off any thoughts, it helps you sleep better and you're also strengthening your bones.

Take time to consider the various forms of exercise readily available to you and decide on one that you can slowly add into your life and one that brings you joy. For you to continue with any form of exercise it's important you enjoy it and look forward to it regularly, it should never be something that causes you anxiety or stress.

Dancing, running, weight training, swimming, yoga, pilates, walking the dog and gardening are all great places to start.

Consider the following when deciding what exercise is best suited to you:

- You enjoy doing it.
- You'll do it long term; it's sustainable and fits into your lifestyle.
- It gives your body a good cardio work out.
- You're physically able to do it, approved by your doctor.

Supplements

Vitamin D

This could well be called the mood vitamin in my view; it's one of the key vitamins needed by the body to maintain balance. As we get older our body's ability to activate vitamin D will reduce, causing a reduction in our ability to assimilate calcium, which in turns leads to an increased risk of osteoporosis, especially in menopause. Vitamin D has a close relationship with calcium, both impacting the brain activity involved in the neurotransmitter processing and the health of the adrenal and pituitary glands. Therefore, if vitamin D is deficient then calcium may lose its power, so it's worthwhile ensuring a diet rich in calcium and vitamin D.

Vitamin D is essential to ensure optimum brain function and we all need to supplement this into our diet every day. For years we have associated vitamin D with stronger bones and teeth (due to its ability to help calcium absorption), it's now well known that vitamin D plays a key role in both sex hormone production (when women are deficient in vitamin D, it reduces oestrogen levels) and mood. A lack of vitamin D diminishes the body's ability to produce feel-good brain chemicals including serotonin and dopamine and as such it's an essential aid to help reduce anxiety.

We can get vitamin D from food sources but we are only able to take a very small proportion of our daily requirement from food. The main food sources are eggs, oily fish, cod liver oil, shitake and button mushrooms and red meat. I would strongly suggest supplementing with an oral vitamin D spray (a higher dose in winter and a lower dose in summer). As vitamin D is an oil soluble vitamin there can be challenges in absorbing it which makes the spray more effective with rapid absorption into the bloodstream.

When next having a blood test, it's worth getting your levels checked as most people these days are deficient in this vital vitamin.

Magnesium

Many of us are now deficient in magnesium no matter how good our diet is and there has been ample research to show the positive effects of magnesium on the nervous system. Modern farming methods in many countries have resulted in the stripping of essential minerals in the soil – with magnesium being one example, so foods grown in magnesium-depleted soil will contain reduced amounts or none at all.

Magnesium is a multi-tasker and plays a part in many processes in the body, from normal muscle function to keeping our bones healthy. Of the many benefits of magnesium, the key one for anxiety is the relationship with GABA, the calming neurotransmitter in the brain. Magnesium can help us relax, it's a key nutrient for the adrenal glands and when we are under stress we actually lose magnesium.

Foods which are good sources of magnesium include:

- wholegrain brown rice
- avocado (one gives you 15% of your daily required magnesium!)
- beans
- nuts
- dark leafy green vegetables like kale, spinach
- quinoa
- oats
- raw cacao powder.

A warm Epsom salt bath at the end of the day will relax your muscles and ensure a deep night's sleep. Personally, I find the powder form of magnesium citrate an excellent sleep aid and easily assimilated by the body.

Calcium

In relation to bone health the key ingredients are calcium, protein, magnesium , vitamin D and vitamin K. These all work in synergy aiding and enhancing absorption of calcium into the bones.

Top foods to eat:

Calcium: milk, yoghurt, cheese, meat, fish, eggs, beans, lentils, fruits (oranges & figs especially), vegetables (go for the greens), nuts and seeds.

Protein: Lean red meat, poultry, fish and eggs are excellent sources of animal protein. Vegetable sources of protein include legumes (e.g. lentils, kidney beans), soya products (e.g. tofu), grains, nuts and seeds.

Vitamin D: oily fish (salmon, sardines and mackerel), eggs, mushrooms and liver.

Vitamin K: another key nutrient for bone health. Vitamin K foods: leafy green vegetables such as lettuce, spinach, cabbage, prunes, liver and soya bean products.

Omega 3

The brain is made up of 60% fat; the encouragement to eat less fat has been turned on its head when it comes to the brain and Omega 3. Of all the oils, Omega 3 is the sacred one, the one that makes your body thrive. Omegas 6 and 9 are more commonly included in modern diets through processing but the healthiest intake comes from avocado, nuts, seeds and rapeseed oil. It requires thought and planning to ensure that you include adequate levels of Omega 3 in your diet. Even when I'm including all the Omega 3 rich foods I can in my diet, I personally feel a supplement is still required. When looking for a good supplement you need to look at the Omega 3 levels of EPA and DHA. EPA is the portion responsible for making neurotransmitters and DHA is responsible for cell building throughout the body.

Good sources of Omega 3 include:

- chia seeds
- flaxseeds
- walnuts
- soyabeans.

Vitamin B Complex

The B vitamins play a vital role in maintaining a healthy nervous system as stress causes depletion. B vitamins are excellent for hair and skin health, in particular riboflavin (vitamin B2) which helps keep skin, nails and hair healthy. Good sources of B2 include milk and eggs. Biotin (vitamin B7) helps the body convert food into energy. It also provides many other benefits including boosting the health of the hair and nails, supporting a healthy pregnancy and helping to manage blood sugar levels.

Food sources

- fish
- eggs

- nuts
- seeds
- A good B complex like Terranova B Complex or Cleanmarine Menomin

Vitamin C

Our adrenal glands, which sit on top of our kidneys, are in charge of the two key stress hormones cortisol and adrenaline, (they also produce oestrogen in smaller amounts). When we are under stress we use our vitamin C supplies up in record time. These supplies are stored in large volumes in the adrenal glands. To ensure optimum health throughout our bodies it's very important to eat foods that are rich in this vital vitamin.

Good food sources of Vitamin C include:

- papaya
- cauliflower
- broccoli
- brussels Sprouts
- blackberries
- strawberries
- kiwis.

Potassium

Potassium is great for your heart health and helps to regulate your blood pressure. Potassium is used by every single cell in our bodies, so if the levels are low you're more susceptible to anxiety and stress.

Good food sources of potassium include:

- avocados
- sweet potatoes
- spinach
- wild caught salmon
- dried apricots (go for unsulfured)
- pomegranate
- coconut water
- banana.

While it might feel overwhelming to overhaul your nutrition and wellness routine completely, a POI diagnosis is often the time to relook at your habits and evaluate the important things that your body may be missing. Even picking just one or two additions or changes to improve your wellness, will go far in supporting you through your POI journey.

Chapter 9

Members' Stories

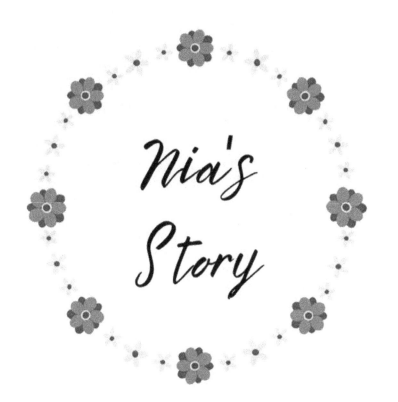

Nia's Story

Hello dear reader. I'm going to compose this as if I'm writing a letter to an old friend so it may seem a little informal. I always find it easier to write as if I'm talking to someone and right now, in this moment, that person is you. I was humbled to be asked if I'd like to contribute to this guide book. I've spoken a couple of times in the past via the wonderful Daisy Network about my experience but was still so honoured to have been approached yet again. This is such a sensitive subject and an incredibly personal one that is unique to each of us. I feel I should mention first and foremost that I understand that the thoughts and processes that have helped me along the way may or may not resonate with you. However, if you can take even a tiny bit of hope from my story or find some semblance of comfort that's wonderful. I know for myself, despite having felt alone and isolated at times, hidden amongst a personal journey such as this one, are common threads that bind us all collectively.

'Journey' there's that word again, a word that seems overused these days. You need look no further than most reality TV competitions. It's also one of my favourite American rock bands but that's a whole other conversation! I love words, they hold such immense power, the words we say to others and equally, if not more important the words we say to ourselves. As you'll soon discover, I love looking up their meaning trying to unearth some new understanding for myself. In an effort to find an alternative word, should 'journey' have lost its impact, I will endeavour to take you on the shorter, less scenic route of my pilgrimage from diagnosis to acceptance.

'Pilgrimage' – noun

A journey, especially a long one, made to some sacred place as an act of religious devotion.

source-dictionary.com

(There's no getting away from the word journey then although I love this substitution. Maybe the sacred place we endeavour to reach is indeed acceptance.)

Part 1 – Shock

I was diagnosed with POI back in 2010 at the age of 35. I wasn't trying for a family, I was single at the time and working in theatre, an industry that seems to keep the ageing process at bay for many. It's certainly not uncommon for women to wait until their 30s or 40s to have a child. Having my own biological child was always something I felt destined to do. It's strange really because that innate knowledge wasn't something I was necessarily conscious of. It's as if it were simply woven into the fabric of my very being.

Early 2009 saw me rehearsing for a new musical, a demanding, often stressful, albeit incredible experience. I was packing up and moving home, sorting through years' worth of memories and in addition to this, my dad was receiving treatment for prostate cancer. So I guess you could say this was a challenging period of time (no pun intended.) My periods disappeared quite suddenly, which I attributed to the stress. Now, despite being quite a warm blooded person, one factor that made me sit up and pay attention was the sweating. Hot flashes, night sweats, these were unnerving and ultimately are what led to me paying my doctor a visit. It really didn't help that the show I was rehearsing was *Sister Act*, this meant hours spent on stage under the hot lights covered head to toe in a habit with only my face and palms exposed. *Wowzers it was hot!* Oh and did I mention that in April 2009 the World Health Organisation declared its first ever 'public health emergency of international concern' in relation to the informally named 'Swine Flu' outbreak (later declared a pandemic). The profusive sweating on the tube to and from work really didn't gain me any admiring glances, with people looking suspiciously at me as if I were sick.

The doctor said that menopause was unlikely given my age but arranged for a myriad of blood tests just to see. Fast forward almost a year and the bombshell was dropped. I was indeed perimenopausal. However, you can still become pregnant during this stage (well I couldn't have without divine intervention but that's beside the point) so there was a glimmer of hope as far as harvesting some eggs. I pinned what little hope remained on the AMH (Anti-Mullerian hormone) blood test. *Were my ovaries still producing eggs and if so, would their quality be good enough?* A few weeks later I received the answer to that question. No.

Tumbleweed, white noise, a really heavy nothingness descended on me literally in that moment. The feeling was palpable and I realised later looking back, it was shock. Complete and utter shock. There's a well-known saying that originates from a famous Chinese proverb – 'A journey of a thousand miles begins with a single step'. I'd love to tell you that my pilgrimage towards peace and acceptance started here but the truth is, I wasn't even close.

Part 2 – Survival

Diary entry March 2010

'Felt very teary at work, I don't want to be there at the moment. I don't want to be home; I just want to be nowhere… floating in space.'

Have you ever had a moment in your life when you know that a shift is ready to happen? Maybe you need to make a huge decision, alter the course you're on. You keep this feeling to yourself, mindful that as soon as you tell someone, speak the words out loud, you've given it energy and brought it to life. From that point it becomes very real and there's no turning back. This has been true for me on more than one occasion but not when it came to my diagnosis.

I opened up to a handful of friends at work, just those who I interacted with most on a daily basis. Telling someone about this devastating news did very little to lessen the weight that I could literally feel on my chest though. They were just words. During those early days and months I had no idea how to accept or even start to process the news and so, I survived. Surviving isn't the same as living, at least it didn't feel that way for me. Getting up, performing daily therefore masking how I felt with another character was my ritual. All the while inside I felt like I couldn't hear myself think, it was just noise and incessant self-deprecating chatter.

The emotional impact of POI was put on the back burner, initially I was just eager to meet with the specialist and gain some further understanding. I had an appointment to discuss HRT and was hopeful that maybe my test results would be explained. None of my peers had been through premature menopause and I was clueless. Even the thought that maybe some medication existed that could jump start my ovaries again crossed my mind.

If I could offer one piece of advice it would be to take someone with you to your appointments. I'd had offers from loved ones but for some reason, I'd already battened down the hatches and decided to go it alone. For a start, I never imagined that the office would be in the maternity unit of the hospital. I had sat waiting amongst pregnant women, how cruelly ironic! I should've at least made some notes but was blindsided by the specialist's demeanour. Just seconds after entering the room I found myself silently reeling at the whole situation. I stepped into his office and was greeted with, 'What can I do for you?'. I realise that the good people who work in the NHS have many patients that they see and of course there's little time for reading notes but still, not even an inkling of why I was there? It threw me for a moment. The conversation soon turned to HRT as it became clear to him that I wasn't in a relationship or actively seeking to have a child at that point. Had that been the case maybe fertility options would've been on the table. What really astounded me was that I could've been seeing him about a common cold. There was zero sensitivity to the fact that I was a woman who had found out just recently that I couldn't conceive. It's not sympathy that you want, just a little empathy and compassion. Nothing was really explained in any detail and I left, still very much confused about why or how this had happened. It turns out there is no reason why for me. There are various factors that can contribute to a premature menopause and then sometimes, it just happens. A random twist of fate.

I'm incredibly fortunate that the HRT tablets prescribed to me seemed to work quite swiftly with no adverse reactions. They helped to lift the cloud around me, steadying my mood somewhat which just left the huge chasm which was the emotional impact.

I can't explain why but I felt like I was less of a woman. As I mentioned earlier, the presumption that I was fertile was somehow naturally present and inextricably linked to who I was as a human being. All of a sudden I was in a tailspin. Flawed, damaged and unworthy I entered into a phase of simply existing. I didn't reach out for help as I couldn't even fathom the idea of looking at how I was feeling. It was as if, in daring to peer over the edge I would fall and then drown in my own sadness. I knew I was sad, deep down in my core but I didn't want to examine that. Family and friends were powerless to help, bless them, it must have been so difficult for those who cared about me. If only I could have found my voice or even sensed how important that was. Every christening or baby shower, Christmas or birthday party I just found myself wanting to retreat. I wish I'd mustered the courage to be able to say, 'I'm struggling today'. Every time I put on a brave face I was stepping in to another layer of emotional clothing. It wasn't long before those layers started to weigh heavy on my heart. Find a dialogue with those closest to you, how else can they possibly understand the magnitude of this diagnosis? It's hard but not impossible and you will feel lighter for it. My lifeline was and still is my best friend and I think it's absolutely vital to have at least one sounding board. Saying that, I can't even remember what we talked about or how articulate I was capable of being. She had just had her baby girl, literally a few weeks after I'd received my news. I had moved and I paid my new doctor a visit. I wanted to ask about some help, some counselling but was met with very little support. Apparently there was someone who visited the surgery every few weeks and they would call me if a slot became available. I didn't get emotional in that meeting. I had already closed myself down so maybe I came across as quite 'together'. Needless to say, I never did get that phone call! As my confidence and self-esteem were pretty much non-existent I didn't even have the nerve to pick up the phone. That task was simply too much for me to even contemplate. The positive news is that there's an abundance of information online now. Blogs and articles that weren't as widely available, if indeed there at all, are now at your fingertips. At the centre of it all, standing strong and true is the Daisy Network thank goodness. Although it was well-established by the time I was diagnosed, sadly I was too busy blocking out my own feelings to even think of delving any deeper or taking advantage of this wonderful resource.

Part 3 – Grief

The element of grief should never be underestimated when it comes to infertility. However, it's incredibly difficult to know how to begin grieving something you never actually had, something intangible. For four years I pushed onwards, simply coping and surviving. I figured I'd managed to learn how to live with what had happened to me but then along came the anxiety. With a heightened heart rate that was pretty constant the weight started to just fall off me. I felt on edge and tears would come at the drop of a hat, seemingly for no reason. *What was happening to me?* I believe our bodies will always manifest how we're feeling and send us signals. Sometimes these nudges are tiny and if we're not aware of them or don't stop to 'listen' they will intensify. It's as if the universe is trying to talk to us. It starts as a whisper and then if we're not getting the message, it will shout! Eventually I heard that shout and I stopped to ask myself why I was feeling this way. Oh boy, then the penny dropped and I just knew instinctively that I hadn't yet grieved. I hadn't grieved for everything that I used to be, everything I thought I would be and everything that I was in that moment back in 2014. I was against the ropes and needed help so I went back to the doctor's practice and saw a different doctor, a lovely man who heard me, really 'saw' me and started the ball rolling with some help of counselling. Unlike the previous appointment I allowed myself to cry, I couldn't keep it inside any longer. It took a few weeks but I eventually started a course of Cognitive Behavioural Therapy (CBT) and had my short-lived experience with seeing a counsellor (a vital service but not the right fit for me).

The edge of grief felt like standing on a precipice and I still didn't know how to step off, it was terrifying. The doctor signed me off work for a while and every night for a week I'd walk up the road from my flat to my best friend's house. She and her husband would feed me and just let me 'be'. I could talk if I wanted but for the most part, I just sat and watched them go about their daily tasks. One evening I was watching a wonderful series on television called *Masterclass*. Hosted by Oprah Winfrey, each episode sees a well-known person, be they an actor, musician, activist, talking straight in to the camera and telling their story. On this particular occasion Jane Fonda was speaking. Partway into the programme she started describing what happens to a muscle when you're working out to make it stronger. She explained how you need to tear the muscle and make it bleed in order for it to repair and strengthen. Then and here is where I literally felt a switch turn on inside me, she likened that to the human spirit. When we are broken, bleeding and we feel at our lowest ebb, there in that moment is an opportunity for transformation. We can repair ourselves and emerge stronger than we were previously. I'd never thought about it that way before. I felt 'less than' because of my diagnosis, I felt weaker, more vulnerable, flawed and damaged. I never stopped to contemplate the possibility that what had happened to me could make me stronger and enable me to be more than I was before. That was it, that was my lightbulb moment. I was still scared as I knew that there was no short cut to take. I couldn't bypass the grief or skirt around it, I had to step off the ledge and move through it. The difference between that moment in 2014 and the previous four years was that

I was ready to feel it, I wanted to feel that sadness. I wanted to get to know the pain that had kept me company for so long, befriend it almost as I knew that was going to be the only way of reaching the other side.

Grief looks very different for each of us and counsel will reveal itself in various ways. There is no wrong or right way, just a way. Mine took the form of writing, reading positive, inspiring material (I'd stayed clear of anything positive for a long time) and sitting under a lot of trees allowing myself to feel. To sit with the pain is essential. If there's one thing I have learned, it's that if we bury our feelings they will only re-emerge again one day. In order not to fear something we have to really expose it and bathe it in light. Keeping it hidden away allows it to remain present. Get it out, look at it, see it for what it's and how it makes you feel, remove the power you've given it and reclaim that power for yourself.

Part 4 – Peace

Time can be a great healer but it doesn't work alone, we have to actively participate in our own healing. As I write this today, I can honestly say that I've made peace with my infertility. When exactly did that happen? I have no idea. There was no gong or whistle signalling the end of my race, no one cheering me on as I took my place amongst the 'I'm doing better' gang. The transformation is quiet and stealthy but powerful none the less. One day I realised I felt ok in social situations that used to make me want to run for the hills. It's entirely possible to feel a genuine happiness for others when they announce their pregnancies as opposed to wishing it could be you. I won't lie though, there is no finish line, I haven't put my feet up knowing the work has been done. I continue to choose peace whenever I can, choosing to feed myself in a positive way whether that means being mindful of what I read/watch/listen to or simply looking away from social media. The moments that floor me, like little punches to my spirit are fewer and fewer these days but they still occur and that's alright. Just a few months ago I watched a toddler navigating his new found mobility and as he fell into the adult's arms I burst into tears. Gone are the days when I would suppress these emotions, now I just ride the waves. What goes up must come down and these moments that move me to my core will always pass if I can just let them be what they are, moments. Please be patient and kind to yourself, anything that requires nurturing needs time and we as human beings are no exception. I only ever wanted to truly feel at peace, not to forget or dismiss such a significant chapter in my life. My infertility will always be part of me, that's non-negotiable but how I choose to live in harmony with it is up to me.

Part 5 – Positively Childless

So what on earth does it actually mean to be 'positively childless'? It sounds so peppy. During the surreal and challenging year that was 2020 I saw so many people using the word 'positive' on almost a daily basis. I understood why and sensed at times that clinging to it in an almost aspirational way was akin to holding on to a life buoy for dear life. When coupled with a friendly nudge of 'don't forget to laugh and have fun' it made me wonder. Do people think that positivity and happiness automatically go hand in hand?

'Positive' – adjective

Full of hope and confidence, or giving cause for hope and confidence

'Hope' – verb

To want something to happen or to be true and usually have a good reason to think that it might

'Confidence' – noun

The quality of being certain of your abilities or of having trust in people, plans or the future

source-dictionary.cambridge.org

None of the definitions above mention the word happy. Think about it this way. A sense of happiness usually arises from another feeling or something quite specific. For example, contentment can lead to happiness but in my opinion, being happy isn't an isolated sensation. It relies on one or more contributing factors. To expect ourselves to just 'be happy' isn't very realistic and can often feel unattainable.

So dear reader, give yourself permission to not always feel happy but endeavour to always search for hope even in the darkest of corners. That hope will look different for each of us, maybe it's about bringing a child into your life through whatever channel is right for you. Maybe, like myself that hope is a simple wish, a prayer for peace deep inside yourself. Keep the faith that wherever your life may take you, you'll be ok. You're ok, you're enough, you're perfectly imperfect as you are!

Nia x

PS What is 'perfect' anyway? Doesn't striving for perfection imply some kind of target, an ideal? I take a lot of comfort from nature, observing the continuous ebb and flow, the constant change and evolution. Aren't we the same? With every passing second we are changing (useful to remember in those dark times when you feel helpless and stuck) and evolving. Our perfection, for want of a better word, may just lie in our imperfections. After all, it's the dents and scrapes, the challenges of life and how we move through them that make each of us a one of a kind original. How perfect is that!

NB If you'd like to get in touch or read about my story in more detail my blogs are available at www. niafisher.com

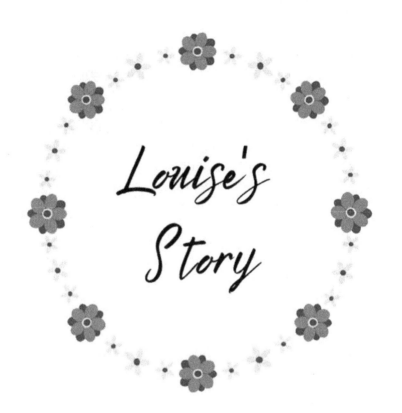

Louise's Story

What a year 2020 was. I was diagnosed with POI in May 2020. It all started when I didn't have a period for four months. I simply thought it was due to stress from a traumatic breakup, and covid causing my dog walking business to turn for the worst.

I've always wanted children of my own, I'm 31 years old. I was concerned that I hadn't had a period for a while. I phoned the doctors in April, they couldn't do anything due to covid, so I had to wait another month before being able to go in for a blood test. Once I had the blood test, I got a phone call two days later from my doctor telling me my FSH & LH were high which meant I had gone into early menopause. My heart immediately sank and I immediately burst into tears, my worst nightmare had become a reality. I couldn't believe what I was hearing. I went into shock, which then quickly turned into anger. I was saying to my doctor, 'This has to be sorted asap. I need to get what is left of my eggs out and frozen.' She told me it didn't work like that and I need another blood test in six weeks' time to confirm the diagnosis. I wanted the second blood test to be done straight away, as I couldn't understand that for an accurate result I needed to wait six weeks.

I felt so angry and upset and kept asking 'why me?' I'm so fit and healthy, the healthiest out of all my friends. I felt so scared and so alone, no one could understand how I was feeling and I just felt I was the only woman suffering from this.

I had no symptoms at all of menopause, only that my periods were absent. I did some research and found I could take an AMH test which tells you if you've a low egg reserve or not. I did the AMH test and it came back as I had the same egg reserve of women who is 45 years old. Hearing this was so hard, I'm 31 this really shouldn't be happening to me.

I wanted to get things sorted asap, so I saw a private gynaecologist who did a transvaginal scan and found that I had five follicles left which was good news, along with that my uterus and endometrial lining was normal and healthy. She then diagnosed me with POI, which I'd never even heard of before. She also said I had a 5–10% of conceiving naturally which will decrease to basically no chance the older I got. I was told about a few different options which include donor eggs, embryo freezing ,egg freezing and adoption. I really wanted to go down the egg freezing route but I had to wait for my second blood test result to come back to see if I was able to go ahead with it or not.

I had so much anxiety over waiting and not knowing what I was going to be able to do. Those six weeks felt like the longest six weeks of my life. I'm single as well, which means it's hard not having a partner to comfort and support me through such a difficult time in my life. I booked myself in with my counsellor to help me and she told me I was going through the grieving process.

I did some research and found there were support groups for women with POI. I joined a couple which helped me knowing that there were other women who are going through it as well. It was great being able to speak to women who could understand exactly what

I was going through. I also found the Daisy Network group, again full of girls/women who understand what having POI is like. For the first time I didn't feel alone.

I had a lot of anger inside of me as us women are only taught about how not to get pregnant and contraception. No one educates you at school, college, university about fertility and fertility problems.

My second blood test result came back with some great news; my levels had dropped by half, which meant I was given the go ahead with trying to freeze my eggs. I was over the moon that I had the option of doing this. Also my periods came back, I had never been so happy to have a period in my life.

I have done one round of egg freezing already. It is the same process as IVF but the eggs are collected and frozen. I had to get over my fear of needles, as I had to inject myself every day with hormones for 10 days. I overcame my fear so quickly and was so proud of myself as that was a massive achievement for me. My first round was a success and I had three eggs frozen. I was literally on cloud nine. Knowing that I will be able to have children of my own in the future when I'm ready, was the best news I had all year. My eggs will always be 31 years old, which means I can have children at any age I want. I'm having two more rounds and am hoping they go just as well as the first one did.

A lot of women who go through this process have a partner by their side for support. I had no one. I know

I had my family and friends but it's just not the same. I know I have always been a strong woman through all the hard times in my life and yet again this has proved to me how strong and how much of a fighter I really am.

I want to now help raise awareness of POI and fertility to others, as I feel it's not spoken about enough and from doing my research, there is little information out there about this. Lastly, for anyone going through this or knows anyone who is, you're not alone; you're strong and if I can do this, so can you.

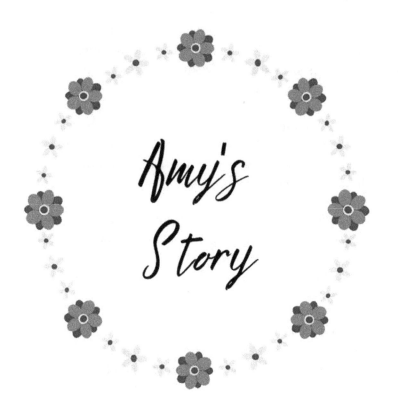

Amy's Story

'Have you started your periods yet?' was a question routinely asked by my mum. My sister started really young at 11 years old and although I was smaller in height than her I think she expected me to follow suit. I was an easily embarrassed kid, so you can imagine my response to being asked this, a red-faced 'no' as I left the room awkwardly. I could understand my mum asking this. I was such a painfully shy quiet child that if I had started my period I wouldn't have even put it past myself to hide it from her. I was always pleased that my answer to the question was no. How embarrassing would it be telling her yes I had started?! I think mums have an intuition too, she just had a feeling that it should have happened by now.

I remember the day my friend was round at my house; we were about to go for a walk to the shops and she quickly went to the toilet before we left. 'Amy, I think I've started my period' she said as she came downstairs looking shocked and a little sick. I went into mother mode, sat her down, made her a cup of tea and gave her a chocolate biscuit for sugar, got a spare pair of underwear and a pad (from my sister's room, obviously not mine) and rang her mum. I handled it like a pro, like someone who dealt with periods all the time, cool as a cucumber, no big deal. Until her mum came over to take her home. 'So have you started your period yet Amy?' an extremely intrusive question to ask a teenager when I think about it now but I reckon due to my age and the way I'd handled helping my friend, she thought I wasn't fazed by it. 'No, I haven't yet' I said sheepishly and she looked surprised. I remember feeling like a failure. This friend was two years younger than me and it was the first time I realised I was falling behind in growing up, I had been overtaken not only by friends my own age but by my younger friends too. I'd never thought of my lack of periods as a problem until then, maybe mum had a point.

When I was 15 years old my mum finally dragged me to the doctors. I'm not going to say I went easily, I kicked up such a fuss because I didn't want to go. Not only was I embarrassed because my doctor was male but also a little bit concerned that something was actually going to be wrong.

'You're only 5ft 2in. That is small for your age. Although 15 years old is late to start your periods. Let's give it another year to see if you're just developing at a slower rate.'

'Super,' I thought 'it's just because I'm small. It will happen in the next year I'm sure of it.' The doctor's appointment seemed to lessen my mum's concerns slightly, knowing that I still had until 16 until it needed to be investigated.

The year passed. I was 16 now, still hadn't grown any taller and still no sign of my period, so once again my mum, with all good intentions, said it was time to go back for investigations.

So after a year of nothing changing, the doctor agreed that it was probably time to do some further blood tests to check my hormones. The phone rang, it was my doctor asking me to go in. I knew that was a bad sign, they only ever ring you if something is wrong.

That's the appointment that changed everything. I went from being a seemingly 'normal' girl who was just a bit small, to being told something that would irrevocably change the course of my life.

'Your blood tests show that your brain is screaming at your ovaries, throwing really high levels of hormones at them to try and make them work and they just aren't responding.' (The doctor even drew a handy little diagram to show me.)

'Will she be able to have children?' my mum asked.

'Not in the traditional way,' the doctor said.

Because my ovaries weren't responding to the hormones, they weren't producing oestrogen, therefore I wasn't ovulating and producing eggs.

I looked over at mum who was now crying. 'What are you crying for?' I asked with a laugh. Whether it was a defence mechanism or whether I genuinely didn't understand the extent of the problem but at that moment I didn't understand the seriousness. I was told I would be referred to a child endocrinologist, who would then sort out my treatment.

I remember going upstairs while my mum told my dad and sister and my sister was upset saying 'I don't understand, she looks so healthy and normal, how can she have something wrong with her and we didn't know?!' I think the news definitely impacted my family more than me. Possibly because it didn't imminently impact my life, having kids was years down the line and I had GCSE's to deal with which was more important for me right at that time. I put the diagnosis in a box in the back of my mind to deal with later. I suppose for my family, they saw the bigger picture. They saw that the reason I was small was due to a hormone issue, that my body wasn't functioning as it should be and that in future, I wouldn't be able to fall pregnant like everyone else. The lack of oestrogen would also have an impact on so many different parts of my body and meant I would be forever battling hurdles as the years went on. It wasn't so easy as just having unresponsive ovaries.

I was referred to a child endocrinologist. At 16 I didn't class myself as a 'child' but in the grand scheme of things, I'm glad in the eyes of the NHS I still was a minor. Having to deal with what was to come would have been worse if it weren't for the doctors specially trained to handle children with care and kindness. The brightly coloured walls and fish tanks did also help as a distraction to the needles.

The first step was to see if they could find the cause of why my ovaries weren't responding. I had blood test after blood test, checking for all sorts of autoimmune disorders and chromosomal abnormalities, ultrasound scans of my pelvis to check I had nothing wrong with my reproductive organs and actually to even check if I had any at all! I remember after the ultrasound scan coming home and saying to my parents that it took so much longer than I expected and I was convinced it was because they couldn't find any organs in there. Just to remind you of what a painfully shy child I was, I wouldn't get changed into my pj's at home without hiding in my bedroom, so getting prodded and poked within an inch of my life in places on my body you can only imagine, just felt so undignified and humiliating. However, all came back clear.

I felt like a freak show. Teen huffiness, mixed with anxiety meant I was pretty snappy and unpleasant in the build up to these appointments.

Why did I get POI? Who knows! After all the tests I had, nothing came back as an identifiable cause, so it has gone down as 'idiopathic', or a medical mystery as I call it. I don't spend too much time dwelling on how or why I have POI, because I can't change it. There's nothing anyone could have done to stop it happening even if we knew the cause.

Surprisingly, one thing I don't feel is sadness or jealousy. I do think about my own fertility at times, like when people around me fall pregnant without even trying, or try once and it immediately happens. I won't have the surprise pregnancy, or the deciding to come off contraception and seeing if and when it happens. It's not that simple for me, that choice has been taken away, but I can't control or change it, so I don't let it cause me any undue upset. *Would I rather I could get pregnant naturally and not have POI?* Well it would make life a lot simpler with a lot less hospital visits but POI has formed who I am today. My adolescence was with POI and my adult years will all be with POI, so it's who I am and I don't know if I would want to be any different. My career path has been formed due to my diagnosis,

I'm now a psychotherapist and my life has purpose as chair of Daisy Network to raise awareness and to help others with this condition. I even have a little tattoo of a daisy on my arm as a proud stamp of what I have been through and how it's a positive part of me.

Through Daisy Network I went from thinking I was the only girl in the country with the condition, to standing on a stage holding a conference surrounded by women with the same thing. If I could, I would show my 16-year-old, newly diagnosed self the image of that room and tell her that she is far from alone and that, yes, it will be tough but you will be ok, in fact, you'll thrive due to POI.

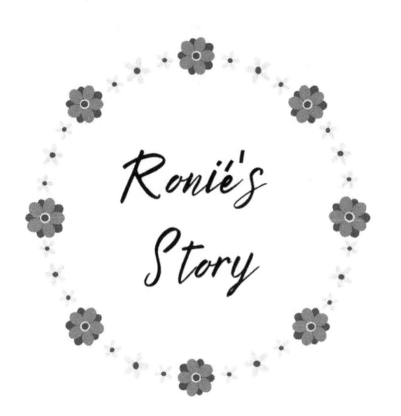

Ronié's

Story

'This is what my mum was talking about,' was my thought as I felt my whole body turn into a ball of flames and tried to concentrate on what my colleague was saying, hoping she wouldn't notice the bead of sweat that was dripping down my forehead.

This was 2015. I was 34 years old. A month before I'd stopped taking my combined pill as my then husband and I decided to try for a baby. We'd been married a year; things weren't great between us but it was the next thing to do right? I'd had cancerous cells removed in my early 20s and the gynaecologist, after removing those naughty cells, assured me 'it's all lovely and pink down there, tubes are all fine, you'll have no problems conceiving'. Phew! Nothing to worry about, I thought. I'd been on the pill since I was around 16 and apart from the issue in my early 20s, had regular periods and didn't even suffer with pre-menstrual tension (PMT) – although I may have got a bit weepy reading a magazine article about a lost puppy on the way to work every now and again. The hot flushes didn't feel great, plus I had a shoulder impingement that was getting on my nerves, so I decided to book an appointment with the doctor and get it looked into.

They sent me for a blood test and a few days later I had a call from the surgery that the doctor wanted to see me. The nice old man, obviously a little bit uncomfortable talking to me about ladies things, bumbled something about something being high and that I needed to be referred for IVF asap if I wanted to think about having a baby. However, I was referred to 'gynae' and was under them for a year. Appointments every three months with a different registrar and never the actual consultant. My periods came and went, came back and went again. Every appointment ended in tears. No real information about what was going on with me. Just asking about my periods and then see you again in a few months. Not even an official diagnosis. Nothing to help keep my spirits up. After no change in a year, we finally were approved for IVF funding and chose Guys as two people I knew had had success there. They were aware of my condition, I'd finally been diagnosed and my husband's sperm count was very low, so it wasn't going to be easy. But they had seen worse. To cut a very long (and at times heart-breaking) story short, we went through the initial cycle; they couldn't regulate my ovaries. I remember one dildo cam scan (my term of endearment for the ultra sound), the doctor just kept saying 'I'm sorry. I'm sorry. I'm sorry,' over and over. I was pulled out of the main part of the fertility clinic into a side room so I could howl in private, with the husband asking me if I'd quite finished. They made an appointment for me to come back and I spoke to one of the amazing doctors there who promised me, that after a few months off the drugs, she'd go in and get the few eggs I had left. As she reminded me, we only needed one good one! However, it wasn't to be. Within three days, my husband and I decided to call it a day, I had to take the IVF drugs back to Guys and that day my nan died. To say the end of 2017 wasn't the best was an understatement. But I was determined to not let life beat me.

I remember vividly the panic attack I had the day I had to take the trigger shot out of my fridge and pack it in to a bag, take a train from where I lived and give it back to the hospital. My only chance of having my own child. I've worked hard at my career since I was 17, however being a mum is the only job I've really ever wanted. I wasn't in a financial position to pursue it alone; my husband had run up debts in the tens of thousands that I knew I would have to clear. My parents offered to pay for me to have the few eggs I had removed but I didn't think I could justify taking their life savings for something that would have no success. I knew I needed to make a big change in my life and so enlisted the help of a psychotherapist and started my CBT/EMDR journey and my pursuit of happiness. I decided that 2018 would be the year I made myself happy. With the help of my saviour and the support of my wonderful family and friends, I managed to dig deep, have blind faith that I could make my life happy again. And I did.

It was the summer of 2018, that I was having some pains and I remembered the cysts that had formed whilst I was going through IVF. At the time I had private medical insurance, so organised to see a consultant to see what was going on 'down there'. I went to see a gynaecologist at the London Bridge hospital, who informed me that maybe I might want to consider going on HRT. Those three letters brought tears to my eyes and brought to mind my mum walking around with a patch on her bum and the adhesive of the ones that had gone before. But I was only 37, surely I didn't need HRT? Surely? She sent me off for another 'dildo cam' over in Harley Street. The lady I saw was amazing. After she'd finished doing her thing, she confirmed I had nothing left in my left ovary and two follicles left in my right ovary. I suffer from osteoarthritis in my neck and shoulders and have two herniated discs that press into my spinal cord. I've had an operation and multiple interventions to try and make it easier for me. And add pain to the rubbish sleep I get most nights. The doctor said I would really benefit from HRT. 'Give it a go, it will make you feel much better', she replied when I told her how upset I was at the thought of going on HRT. I had also just met someone new, five years younger than me. I didn't want him knowing I had to take HRT. Or see a patch on my bum, or the remnants of, when it was time to, well you know… Imagine him waking up one day with my patch stuck to him and having to explain that away. The thought made my toes curl. But I decided to give it a go. The gynaecologist prescribed an HRT that unfortunately was no longer available and then I was given Elleste Duet to try and to go back to see her in a month. I remember picking up my prescription from the chemist and being charged £16 for one prescription. 'Erm, excuse me, I don't think that's right'. The poor pharmacist had to explain that it's a double charge because of the two different pills in the pack. 'Well, isn't this the gift that keeps on giving, it's bad enough I have to be on HRT at my age but now I have to pay twice for the privilege,' I muttered as I tapped my debit card. The dark mood and black cloud that began to follow me wouldn't shift. I felt so sad and down all the time. I was, admittedly still going through separation and having therapy and my psychotherapist told me about calcium and magnesium supplements and how they had helped her with her PMT. They really helped balance my mood but HRT really wasn't working for me. I called Bupa to get follow up with my doctor but was informed that as I had been prescribed HRT they deemed my problem to be 'age related' and they wouldn't cover me going forward. Age related at 37!!! I couldn't afford to see her privately and she didn't see anyone through the NHS but her secretary suggested I speak to my doctor and be referred to the early menopause clinic at Guys. I managed to speak to my doctor who was incredibly understanding and suggested I went back on the pill I used to be on previously, as I never had a problem with it but this time round it just gave me a continuous bleed. I managed to get into the clinic a few months later and spoke to a fantastic doctor who finally explained much more about POI. It was her specialist subject and was looking to do more research on why it happens. She said she'd send me through to the specialist POI team and I would be under their care going forward. Praise be! Finally, I felt that I was being taken care of.

I've now been on HRT for just over two years. I've worked my way through six of them; with all the side effects, moods, acne, weight gain (my particular favourite – almost two stone). Despite having a personal trainer, being very active and having a calorie-controlled diet for two years, I've not been able to shift a pound. I decided to come off Femoston 2/10 for a while to see; I didn't have any menopausal symptoms before I went on HRT, surely I'd be fine?? Wrong – full body flushes, heart palpitations, lying awake for hours. I lost 2kg in two weeks but I clearly need the oestrogen. I have recently had the coil fitted and top it up with oestrogen gel, so we'll see how that goes. I'm waiting for the flashbacks of the fitting to leave me and for my private parts to feel normal again. Oh and the acne. I'm told there's acne. Yay! (I told you it's a gift that keeps on giving.)

I know I am luckier than most. I'm in the system. I get 15 mins of the menopause clinics' time every six months. It's something... I have a great support network. A close, loving family; kind and caring friends and colleagues and a lovely boyfriend. He has two children and I am loving getting to know them. I had to recalibrate when they first met my parents. It was wonderful and heart breaking at the same time. I know they would hate it but the guilt I feel for not being able to give them grandchildren will never leave me. And sometimes despite all this I can often feel totally alone. Because try as they might; my best friends, even my mum can't understand some of the feelings I have. They have all the hormones they need; at the time they need them. They have their children's unconditional love.

That's where the Daisy Network comes in. I have been having an incredibly hard time over the last six months. I mean who hasn't? I have the propensity to over work, as I don't have that 'other commitment' to bring me back to what's important in life. I am a person where work defines me. It's what I have poured my everything into, even my soul at times. My osteoarthritis went into overdrive and I've been in excruciating pain. Too many inputs, not enough filtering out. I remembered about Daisy and posted on a SE London forum. A wonderful lady got back to me and said how I was feeling resonated with her and asked if I wanted to be added to a WhatsApp group of other Daisy members. Yes I did. Because to be in the company of someone who knows how I feel would be great. They might have a different story but they will know that sometimes you just don't feel well at all. That sometimes you just want to cry. They know that sometimes life feels so unfair. And you're angry and wonder why this had to happen to you. They just know and you don't have to apologise about feeling it or saying it, or feel like they're going to pity you. They just know. A few of us met up for a walk just before the last lockdown and it was fun and informative. four women, walking round a park with a coffee, talking about fannies and dildo cams and HRT like it was normal. Because it is. The big 40 is approaching next year. I want to make the years count. I want to do more for o ur community, in any way I can. Thank you, the Daisy Network, for existing. For allowing me to tell my story. If there is anyone struggling out there who needs a chat, please get in touch.

Ronié

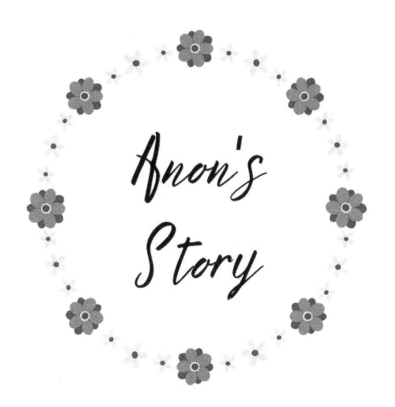

Anon's
Story

As a British Asian Muslim raised within a strict household, my early menopause was firmly diagnosed around age 16 years.

Today, I am nearing a milestone to half of my life and writing this still leaves me with a heavy heart and questions of how my life would have been with children or who I really am.

I have cried, reflected and ultimately been in denial as being childless with Asian communities was seen as taboo and approaching the topic was as awkward as a first date!

There are prominent words in almost every Asian girl's day-to-day life like Sharam (embarrassment/shame) and Izzat (honour/reputation). These words followed me throughout my journey. I think the impact upon my parents was the greatest as they carried the burden of denial and regret which they could never express.

As the years crept on I dreaded family and community functions which revolved around the topics of a suitable boy, marriage and children mirroring the Indian movies.

I became the artful dodger with an excuse, witty joke or selective hearing to protect the sadness in my mum's eyes.

Rising through university to a working professional, I have seen my family and friends welcome the joy of children through their journeys.

Today I feel I have accepted my place in society which does not conform to traditional values of Asian society. Upon reflection, I feel the stars were not aligned for me to have children as I may not be who I am today.

My family, friendship, connections through the Daisy Network and being true to myself is the biggest gift and oasis.

I hope a new generation will dismiss the taboo topic of early menopause and ease the feelings of embarrassment, reputation, shame and culture which I experienced.

Today I smile when hearing the strength from Asian women wanting to discuss, seek support and challenge the stigma with confidence and inner beauty.

Love, anonymous x

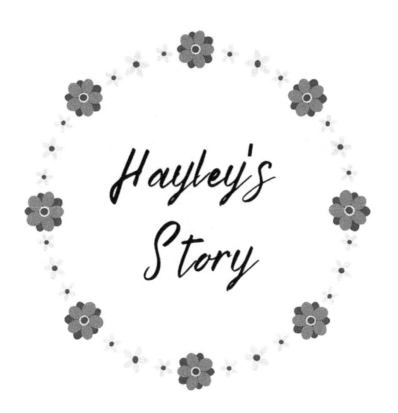

Hayley's Story

I was 14 years old when I was told I had gone through the menopause... yep that's right 14 years old.

I will never forget that day, sitting on the bed in a hospital room waiting for the consultant to come to me and my mum saying those words. My mum balling her eyes out and me comforting her asking her to not cry as it's ok. Thing is it wasn't ok but then I had no clue what the consultant was even talking about.

At the age of 12 I started my periods like a normal teenager. Then after a year they just stopped. I was struggling to concentrate at school and the nights were hell. Waking up dripping with sweat and just feeling weird. That's literally how I described it to my mum one day. I don't feel like me mum, I feel weird. So off we went to the doctors. I explained what was going on and I was referred for a blood test and an ultrasound. Then two weeks later a consultant gynaecologist confirmed I had gone through my menopause and that I needed to start taking HRT tablets.

I was told I had a uterus but a small one and that they could only find one ovary. That was the first and the last time I was going to see my consultant. I am now 39 years old. I literally have never been contacted since. Not given any follow-up appointments, no help, no guidance to understand what had happened to me, nothing. Put on Prempak C and left to just get on with it.

Even when Prempak C was discontinued a few years back I wasn't even informed by my doctor. The pharmacist told me when I went to pick up my meds.

Meds, may I add that I have to pay for... which I find astonishing. I need to take these daily and I had none left so luckily after a long phone call I managed to get in with a doctor the next day. Who then told me there was no exact alternative and she was putting me on another brand. But that was horrendous. All my levels went crazy and my symptoms returned and my bleeds were so painful. I then was changed onto Femoston which I now take and luckily have no problems with. Even my bleed isn't as painful anymore as I have to have one monthly to keep the lining of my uterus working properly, in-case I was to decide I wanted to try IVF. Something I have decided against, as I cannot go through a grieving process again if it wasn't successful.

As a child I needed to learn what it all meant and back then there was hardly anything on the internet to read and even to this day limited material to a teenager experiencing this happening to them. This needs addressing as I felt lost for years as I just didn't understand it all. Medical professionals looked at me like I was some sort of freak. If I was given a pound for the amount of times a doctor or nurse has said to me you poor girl when I answer the dreaded question... 'what medication do you take'. I would have had loads of work done on myself. Which leads me on to how I have felt growing up... hating what I saw looking back at me in the mirror. The one job a woman is given to do and I couldn't even do that properly. I felt like a failure. A failure as a woman.

I can't say I grew up depressed I just learnt how to cope. I grew up not liking my appearance. I suppose

I felt insecure about myself. I struggled with relationships with guys as I knew I had it looming over me that one day I was going to have to tell them. Even when I did tell them or my friends neither understood. I even lost a friend over it as she said I was lying and that it was a sick thing to make up! Charming! The response I got from the close few I did tell was always the same... 'It will happen one day mate, loads of women are told they can't have kids and they do'.

Nobody understood what I was saying. Because no one was/is educated enough. No one knows what it means. Even to this day people still do not understand. So, in my words I say it how it is... . To produce a baby, you need an egg and a sperm and I don't have eggs, end of.

Literally one week ago I decided I was ready to talk about my experience out loud and to try and get this recognised more. To get people to speak out and not hide it all inside, because you feel everyone will be gossiping about you.

Unfortunately, it happens to all of us females one day. There is no set age limit on it, which I am living proof of.

My journey to become a Mum...

For me I decided that egg donation was not the route I wanted to go down to become a mummy.

I think because I found out at such a young age (14), I had grown up accepting that I was never going to biologically have my own child and thought I would rather adopt a child than try IVF.

I also worried that maybe I would struggle emotionally knowing that our child would be half of my husband and may even feel jealous of that at times.

Adoption in my mind was always going to be the way and I made this very clear when I told my husband about my premature menopause and what it meant regarding becoming parents.

Maybe I was being selfish denying him of being a biological father but that's where I was wrong.

Gavin's mum was in fact adopted so for him adoption was not a taboo subject and he had grown up knowing his whole life of adoption. His grandad was his absolute idol and it didn't matter about blood relation to him. He knew it was more about love.

Back in May 2020 during the first covid lockdown, we decided we were ready to make that call to find out about beginning the adoption journey. We felt so excited that we were finally at the right stage in our lives to now grow our family and we were ready to put our hearts and souls into it, to achieve that dream.

It is tough I won't lie but when you're ready you just get through it. There is lots and I mean lots of paperwork to get through. You've three stages which are the pre-stage, stage 1 and then stage 2.

The pre-stage – after making that first enquiry you receive forms to fill in and then they make the decision if they would like you to attend an information meeting. You then have more forms to complete and depending on whether they are happy you get accepted into stage 1.

That's when the hard work begins. You have to attend several training days, complete a first aid paediatric training course, pass medicals, references need to be given (with replies), complete a chronology of your whole lives and really go into depth in certain areas. Alongside this you've to do reading, watch things and just learn, learn, learn. Your social worker will then decide if she thinks you're suitable and ready to be accepted into stage 2 and will give their recommendation to their manager who makes the final decision.

I am happy to saw we have recently been accepted into stage 2 and should be starting anytime soon. This will be when your social worker basically becomes your therapist and will get to know us probably more than anyone else. They will go through your lives in detail, how you dealt with certain situations see what kind of child you would be best suited for.

We have chosen to adopt a child between the ages of 0–4 years. We do not mind whether it's a girl or a boy. Just as long as they are healthy.

Stage 2 will also consist of further training days and our social worker will get us prepared for panel to become approved adoptive parents.

The time frame really is not as long as you would think from the initial enquiry to becoming approved. So, don't let that put you off. I would say a year maximum.

The time frame to get to panel once in stage 2 is 16 weeks so I like to think by June we will be approved, so wish us luck!

If anyone would like to ask me anything regarding the adoption process, please feel free to give me a shout... x hayleysmenopause14.blogspot.com

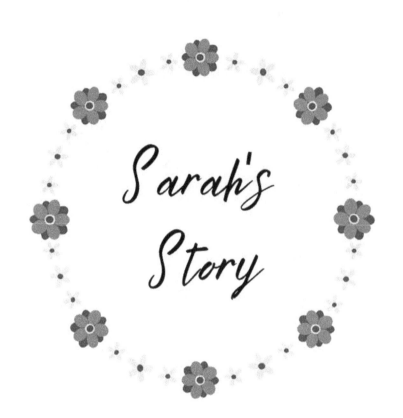

Sarah's Story

I had just completed my postgraduate studies at university when my POI symptoms started. I was single, in my mid 20s and embarking on a career that is often viewed as demanding and stressful. I suffered from horrendous migraines, which were always followed with vomiting episodes because the pain was so great. I also felt extreme tiredness and anxiety.

I went to the doctor many times but was told that it was the stress of my profession that caused this and that it's normal. 'Take it easy,' was my prescription. After repeated visits, I was offered antidepressants although I never took them; the rational part of me knew that I was not depressed. It was very frustrating. When my periods stopped, I begged the doctor to send me for tests. Coming from a broken home, I always wanted a family, so I was desperate to find out if my fertility was ok. The doctor told me that since I was only 30, I was 'ridiculous' to worry and it was most likely the stress of my profession causing the amenorrhea. After repeated begging, my doctor reluctantly agreed to send me for tests. I will never forget the results day. As I cried all I could say was, 'Who will love me now?' I felt broken, unlovable and no longer a 'real' woman.

I am sure I suffered PTSD from the experience of such devastating news. I was not offered any counselling, time off work or follow up support.

The diagnosis has affected my confidence in relationships with men. I have been broken up with because I cannot give my own children. I also suffer with health anxiety and presume the smallest ache or pain must be something terrible.

POI has impacted my life hugely– but most effects cannot be seen by others. It is as though I have no illness and therefore, I have little support, compassion or understanding. Over the years, whenever I tried to confide in other women about POI, I have been told that it's not possible and that my diagnosis must be wrong. If I say that I am struggling with tiredness, aches, or pains, I am compared with other women my age, so I have been made to feel lazy or unmotivated. It is evident that even friends that know about my condition struggle to believe me because my symptoms are not visible. Consequently, I stopped mentioning it at work or to friends. I have never wanted pity, just understanding.

The journey to being diagnosed and the following years show the lack of awareness that doctors and the public have about this condition.

The Daisy Network has been a tremendous help in providing information and support. I am so happy about the work they are doing to spread awareness of this condition. I have made wonderful friends who have been understanding and supportive. My hope for the future is that there is more training and a wealth of information available for doctors to help diagnose and support young women with this condition.

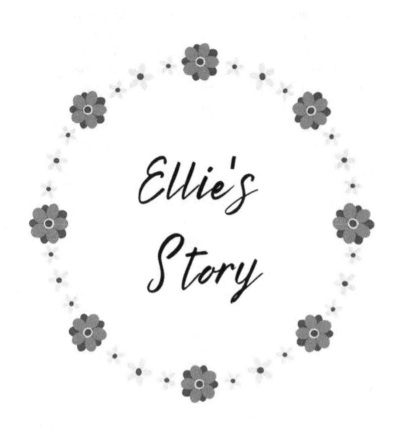

Ellie's Story

Unlike most, my POI diagnosis was expected. It was a side effect of my cancer treatment.

When I was 14 years old, I was diagnosed with a rare childhood cancer, called Alveolar Rhabdomyosarcoma. To combat the cancer I had to undergo 18 months of chemotherapy and 28 sessions of pelvic radiotherapy. I am currently three and a half years into remission and remain cancer-free – whoop whoop!!! But unfortunately, cancer doesn't end when treatment finishes. I am left with a myriad of long-term side effects, the most prominent being infertility. The chemotherapy caused my ovaries to stop functioning properly, so I went into early menopause. And, on top of that, the pelvic radiotherapy scarred my uterus, damaging it so much that even carrying a baby is impossible for me.

When the doctors told me that the treatment would make me infertile, I honestly wasn't that bothered. I was in survival mode. So, all I could focus on was beating the cancer and I was determined to do whatever it took. It wasn't until about three months into remission that I allowed myself to start thinking about the future again, which led me to become more curious about my fertility and lack of it. So, I asked my consultant, 'on a scale of one to ten, with one being not very fertile and ten being very fertile, how fertile am I?' She replied, 'zero'. I don't know why I asked her this as I knew deep inside what the answer was already but I guess part of me hoped that because I defied the odds of surviving my cancer, I would also defy the infertility diagnosis and prove my doctors wrong. That consultation didn't make me feel sorrow or grief, instead it made me determined to accept the diagnosis and embrace it – I survived cancer, so I wasn't going to let infertility bring me down.

The first time I heard someone mention the word 'menopause' I was about six months into remission and I informed my consultants that my periods had not returned. They ran a series of blood tests to discover that my FSH levels were through the roof and my oestrogen levels were barely existent, leading to the diagnosis of POI. Again, I wasn't too bothered about the diagnosis. I had overcome many much larger obstacles so POI seemed fairly insignificant to me. And, I must admit, that I was fairly elated by the prospect of no periods. But I would soon come to realise that POI was going to be one of my biggest challenges yet.

As far as I was aware, the menopause meant no periods and that was all but what my consultants failed to tell me was the other consequences of the menopause, such as fatigue, achy joints, vaginal atrophy and brain fog. So, I was suffering with these horrendous symptoms, thinking they were late effects of the chemotherapy but they were actually due to the menopause!! My consultants put me on HRT but at that time, I didn't realise that HRT dosages can vary and that teenagers should have a much higher dose than the average menopausal women. Consequently, I suffered with menopausal symptoms for way too long. Even my doctors didn't think the problems I were having were due to my oestrogen deficiency.

At a time when I should have been happy that I had survived cancer, I felt down and irritated by the huge burden of my cancer treatment. I felt like I was 18 going on 80. Whilst my peers were out doing part-time jobs, pursuing intimate relationships and going to parties, I was in bed by 10pm each night and was disgusted by the very thought of having a boyfriend – being a single cat lady for the rest of my life seemed perfect to me. I knew this wasn't how I was meant to feel as a teenager but I didn't know how to fix it. This made me feel like a complete outsider, which really affected my self-confidence. But, as usual, I carried on and distracted myself by excessively studying for my A-levels. I should've told someone how I was feeling but I didn't feel that I was able to. As a cancer survivor, I should be appreciative of the simple fact that I am not dead, so I felt too guilty to complain about such trivial problems such as fatigue, low sex drive and vaginal pain. This meant that I suffered in silence for months on end.

The turning point for me was lockdown. Overnight, I suddenly had no school work to distract me, so my only focus was myself. Therefore, the issues I had been burying under the sand for so long suddenly became much more profound. So, for the first time, I was forced to deal with my issues head on as I knew I could not live in this dire existence for much longer. Moreover, lockdown brought a completely new problem: a boy. At a cancer event I attended the previous year, I had met an amazing guy, we stayed in contact and, as much as I tried to suppress the feelings, it was becoming clear to me that I liked him much more than just a 'friend'. So, for the first time in forever, I was actually considering an intimate relationship with someone. But this imaginary fairy tale came crashing down by the harsh realisation that I had no sex drive whatsoever, my clitoris no longer worked and my vagina felt as dry as the Sahara desert. I knew I couldn't live like this anymore. I wasn't going to let these issues dictate the rest of my life. I wanted a future with a husband, children and much more, so I knew that if I didn't act then I would never live the life I wanted to. It made me realise that I didn't have to feel guilty about complaining – remission isn't sunshine and rainbows. I realised that I have got to live the rest of my life in this body so it's up to me to get it fixed.

Realising that this problem wasn't going to fix itself, I decided to do my own research. From listening to Dr Newson's podcasts and reading Jane Lewis's *My menopausal vagina*, I became empowered with knowledge about how the menopause can affect all different parts of your body, allowing me to gain insight into what my body needed. Since finishing treatment, I felt so out of control with my menopausal symptoms but suddenly I felt like I had some control back and I was excited to share this knowledge to get the best treatment for myself. From the research I did, I knew that I would like to have my oestrogen medication increased, some local oestrogen for the vaginal dryness, a DEXA scan to check my bone health and a prescription of testosterone to get my sex drive back. Armed with all of this knowledge, I went to see an NHS endocrinologist and confidently told him what I thought was best for me but I came out of the appointment extremely underwhelmed as the only action he wanted to take was to increase my oestrogen dose from 20mcg to 30mcg, leaving the addition of local oestrogen for a later date.

I didn't want to wait. At this time, waiting felt torturous, I had already been battling with my declining emotions about the state of my menopause, so the only way I was going to feel happy was to get the medication that I needed. So, I decided to go private.

'Hi. My name is Ellie, I would like to book an appointment with Dr Newson.'

The receptionist said, 'Of course, how old are you?'

I replied, 'I am 18 years old.'

There was a huge pause before the receptionist asked, 'Are you sure you've the right number?'

That moment made me realise how alone I was, if even a menopause clinic hadn't come across a teenager with the menopause, then what hope did I have of meeting others in the same situation as me?

A half-hour conversation with Dr Newson accomplished more than had been done in the three years since I finished treatment. She reassured me that she would help to get my symptoms under control and she prescribed everything I asked for as she had the same notion as me that it's best to throw everything at it and make you feel better sooner. It felt like a huge relief to finally get the help I needed.

Making the decision to seek menopause care privately is the best decision I have ever made. Whilst I am forever grateful for the NHS and all of the life-saving treatment it provided for me, I feel the endocrinology and menopause services are severely lacking. For three years since being diagnosed as menopausal, the HRT I received was inadequate and I never saw an actual specialist, so I was left in the dark, too afraid to voice my issues, as I felt like I was going to be disregarded. But now I realise that the delay in getting the right menopause care massively affected my physical and mental wellbeing, ultimately hindering my cancer recovery. Ever since being on the new HRT regime, I have improved leaps and bounds. It amazes me to see how I went from a very insecure, unhappy person to where I am now: full of energy, confidence and hope for the future.

The best thing that has come out of all of this is the people I have met along the way. Before, I felt like the only teenager in the world who was going through the menopause. But, since sharing my story on YouTube, I have come across many other teenagers in the same situation as me; it feels amazing that I am able to talk to them if I ever need some support or advice. Moreover, sharing my menopause story has led to fantastic opportunities. I have been on podcasts and Instagram lives talking about my POI journey – I have even spoken openly about my vaginal issues, which I would have never done a year ago! It feels great that I can use my story to spread awareness and help other girls in the same situation as myself. Most excitingly, I am working with Dr Newson to write a booklet for young women with cancer who are going through the menopause. I am so happy to have met Dr Newson and have this amazing opportunity, because this booklet is exactly what I wished I had three years ago when I was diagnosed. It feels great that I am part of a community that is so passionate to spread awareness of POI and improve the services provided to these young women.

The Daisy Network has been instrumental in my POI journey because they made me feel accepted when I felt most alone. Being able to go on their Facebook group and chat to others who know exactly what I am going through was very therapeutic for me. And being able to attend workshop sessions about unspoken topics, such as POI and sex, really changed my attitude about myself. Before I felt undesirable but now I embrace my POI, I will never hold myself back from pursuing a relationship again. What I have realised is that POI is a very small part of me and should not define my life going forward. I am very hopeful for the future and no longer feel like an outsider. For the first time since my cancer diagnosis, I feel normal again.

Ellie x

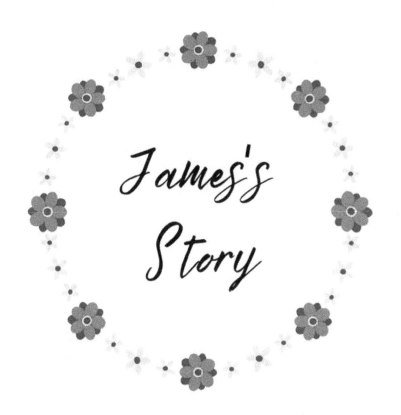

James's Story

I will never forget the look on Holly's face the day she was diagnosed with POI. The usual sparkle in her eyes had gone. With a shaky voice, while trying to hold back the tears, she explained the scan had shown her ovaries had shrivelled and there were no visible eggs left. The doctor had told her she wouldn't have her own children and IVF was not available on the NHS as it was unlikely to work.

By now the tears had broken free and were streaming down her face as she offered me a way out of our marriage. Six short months ago we had the best day of our lives when we said 'I do' in the south of France in the blazing sunshine surrounded by lavender, olive trees and our nearest and dearest. We had written our own vows which were beautiful, loving and unique to us, however we didn't actually promise 'for better, for worse, for richer, for poorer, in sickness and in health'. Holly went on to say she loved me and because she loved me, she wanted me to be happy and have the most wonderful life possible. She couldn't see this for herself then and quite matter-of-factly she said, 'This isn't what you signed up for and if you want to leave I totally understand and support your decision with no hard feelings'. Without hesitation I gave her a massive bear hug and answered, 'No way, we are in this together, through the good and the bad, all the highs and the lows!' We made a pact that day that together we would take on anything POI throws at us and we wouldn't give up the life and children we always dreamed of.

Neither Holly nor I had heard of POI before her diagnosis, we were keen to find out more and meet others who were going through the same challenges. I took charge by taking to Google and I came across the Daisy Network. They are a fantastic charity who provides a focal point for women with POI and their partners to get support throughout their journey as well as to raise public awareness of the condition. We were fortunate that they had an event, the Daisy Day, coming up soon. I jumped straight in and bought us tickets. Initially Holly didn't want to go; I think she was worried she may not be able to go without crying in public but after some persuading she was in.

I arrived at the first day of Daisy Day on my own, Holly was coming a couple of hours late after work. I was pleasantly surprised to see so many men there with their partners. Their commitment and bravery to attend blew me away and I realised immediately that we were not alone and I was optimistic that we would find the help and community we were searching for.

At the first morning talk I was keen to highlight that Holly was arriving later and that she was newly diagnosed and we were both struggling. I asked everyone if they would kindly say hello to Holly when she arrived and offer any words of wisdom they may have. I must say the support was overwhelming! It was amazingly uplifting for me to see so many women exchanging mobile numbers and giving Holly healing hugs. I was also able to chat to men in the same boat as me and to this day we have kept in contact and we continue to support each other on this unique path.

Following Daisy Day, Holly and I were high off hope. We came to realise that the doctor was wrong, we could still have our own children through egg donation or adoption. With couples and individual counselling along with sharing our situation with our community we slowly let go of the vision of life we thought we would have to make space for what was to come (which can still be incredible).

After researching all avenues we decided donor egg IVF would be the way we would like to grow our family. We decided to pursue this in Prague, Czech Republic. The IVF process is certainly a rollercoaster ride of ups and downs. So far we have had two transfers which unfortunately both were unsuccessful. There have been many tears plus the grief to process but we are not giving up on our dream.

Throughout our experience, as a husband, it took me a long time to accept that I could not simply make everything better for my darling wife – it was extremely hard to stomach. I struggled at times to communicate effectively with her because I felt like I was walking on eggshells as I didn't want to say the wrong thing and upset her when she was already in so much pain. I think daily walks after work were the key, being out of the house and in nature together it was easier to find the right words. As we kept talking it became clear Holly didn't want me to tell her 'everything is going to be ok'. She wanted me to show her I wasn't going anywhere and I would be next to her to hold her up no matter what. So I vowed I'm not going anywhere, I'll be there whether she wants me to be or not!

Four years on POI is still very much part of our lives, be it travelling to London for medical appointments, grieving the loss of unsupportive friends, running around Prague trying to find french fries and a pineapple to help our embryos 'stick' or investigating the right kind of lubrication. It's been a bumpy but transformative adventure. Holly and I truly aren't the same people we were before this happened – we are far more kind, compassionate and open-minded, I think we'll be better parents when we get there too. We have honestly found out what matters to us in life. Holly has become even more beautiful inside and out. I'm in awe of the strength she has cultivated to take the cards she has been dealt and run with them. She worries she is viewed as a victim but it's the absolute opposite that she is a warrior and an inspiration.

Looking back it's unbelievable what we have navigated and survived as a couple. Holly has the sparkle back in her eyes and our relationship is stronger than ever. We are now diving into our third IVF cycle and we can't wait to meet our rainbow baby... Wish us luck!

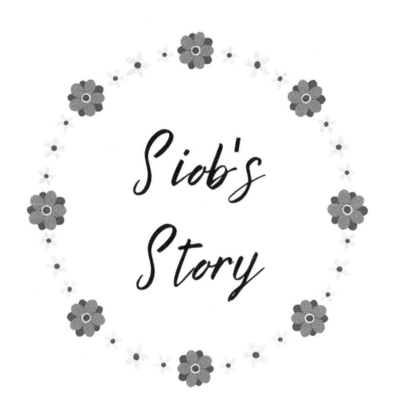

Siob's
Story

I have been a stay at home mum since my daughter was born (she was conceived on donor egg IVF round number three then we went on to do another unsuccessful fourth round when she was 16 months old). I was looking for the next step in my life once she started school. I considered returning to nursing, trying out an entirely new career, going back to university. I even entertained the idea of a new puppy or getting a sports car. There was an itch that I needed to scratch, I just couldn't find it.

While trying to conceive I remember feeling there was no way I could adopt. I couldn't stand the idea of a social worker coming into my home and my life, asking questions and judging me. Especially when I knew in my heart I'd be a good mum. But one afternoon before preschool pick up, out of nowhere, the idea of adoption popped into my head and I couldn't shake it. I spoke to my husband about it and he wasn't keen. We had only just become financially stable again after all the IVF. We were settled as a family of three.

I asked him to come to an information evening in November with the social services adoption team. It was very informal and previous adopters gave short talks about their experiences. To say we were underwhelmed would not be an exaggeration. We decided more or less in the car park it wasn't for us.

Christmas is a sentimental time of year. We were both a bit sad watching our daughter opening her presents by herself. At the time she had no cousins and there were little prospects of any coming. We talked on Boxing Day and decided we'd go for it.

The process started very quickly in January. After our first meeting with our assigned social worker, she advised us that we should start telling everyone in our lives about our plans because we could have a child placed with us within six months. In reality, things took a little longer than that. We were approved adopters by that December and our son moved in with us the following May aged six months old.

Life as a family of four has been a big adjustment. I'm a lot more tired now than I was the first time around. My son is three now and he is such a pickle! He's a lot more active than my daughter. And he's so cheeky! But he has the most beautiful grin and gives the biggest hugs. He makes my heart swell. I love him so much, I'm so proud I get to be his mummy.

I think about the future and how being adopted might affect him. After all, he wasn't given up for adoption, he was removed from his birth family. That is something he will grow up knowing and we'll navigate it together. But I know I love him; he's the best little whirlwind life has thrown at us. Even his big sister is smitten... most of the time!

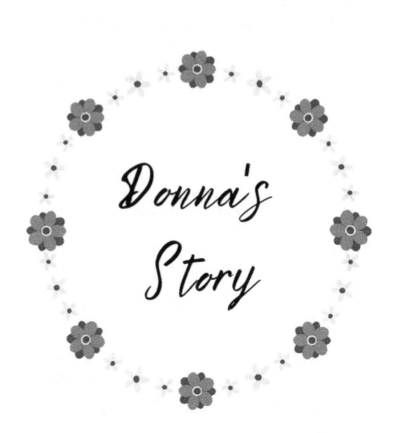

Donna's Story

Looking back, I distinctly remember the moment my peri-menopause symptoms started at the age of 29, although I had no clue what was happening to me at the time. I just felt a kind weird shift inside me on both a physical and mental level, my heart was pounding, my face and neck were bright red and I felt completely panicked and short of breath. Not long after this, my periods disappeared for a year and a half. On separate occasions, I visited my doctor for what I thought was anxiety disorder and also for my lack of periods.

Regarding the anxiety, my doctor told me to save some money and go see a private councillor as I probably wouldn't get the time off work to see an NHS therapist anyway. As for my missing periods, my bloods were tested (I was not told what they were tested for) and I was referred to University College Hospital for an ultrasound. The nurse told me that there was no sign of ovulation. I left my appointment and was never contacted by the hospital or my doctor regarding this again. For the next few years, I just carried on as normal, periods would come and go and the anxiety got even worse, social situations began to trigger what I thought were panic attacks but looking back now, they were actually intense hot flushes spiralling out of control.

By the time I was 34, my periods stopped completely and that's when things got bad with my mental health. I could barely communicate with people as it would trigger my panic attacks. I avoided social situations and my career suffered as my managers couldn't understand my lack of confidence. I would sit freezing in vests and t-shirts in cold air-conditioned offices, not daring to put a jumper on as I was terrified to overheat and trigger the redness and panic attack. I went back to my doctor and was referred to talk therapies and given beta blockers, neither of which made any difference.

Things came to a head at the age of 37 when I visited my gynaecologist due to my copper coil causing me immense pain. Much to both our complete shock, the device had dislodged itself (the cervix shrinks in menopause) so she removed it and then asked when my last period was. She then suggested I go to my doctor for an FSH test as I could be in early menopause. I was absolutely horrified. I had no idea how the menopause would affect my health at that point, it was more the stigma of it that bothered me then. Little did I know, that would be the least of my problems.

A week after my FSH test I hadn't heard anything, so I telephoned my doctor for the results, the receptionist picked up and responded by saying 'I have them here, yes, you're menopausal'. I asked when the doctor wanted me to come in and receptionist told me that there was no note to say he wanted to see me. I put the phone down. At this point I had never felt so alone in my life... but then I found the Daisy Network.

My doctor told me he thought menopause shouldn't be a big deal for me as I was in my late 30s anyway. He also told me that HRT increased the risk of cancer, so I found a consultant with some POI knowledge who gave me HRT and referred me for a bone scan. Unfortunately, I was diagnosed with full blown osteoporosis and then went on to break my ankle in a climbing accident a month later. My doctor attempted to refer me to the orthopaedic consultant at the local hospital however he refused to see me as he felt that osteoporosis is normal for menopausal women (I was 38 at this point). From then on, I decided to become my own doctor and empower myself to take charge of my own wellbeing. Obviously, I grieve for the children I will never have. I've had to give up things I love such as snowboarding and climbing but two years after my diagnosis I am now the best version of myself. I have my off days but most of the time I am loving life and still excited for what else is to come. I know I have so much to offer and that I am more than enough, even as a woman that can't have children. I can't change my ovaries but I have learned to heal myself on a spiritual, mental and emotional level. My career is going well, I have a collection of knitted jumpers that I can wear without a second thought and I have switched snowboards and climbing walls for sailing, which gives me the adrenaline rush I need without the impact on my bones. Whether you're 15 or 51, menopause is not the end of your life, it's just the beginning of a new chapter. My biggest lesson from all this is that you can't control the wind but you can adjust the sails.

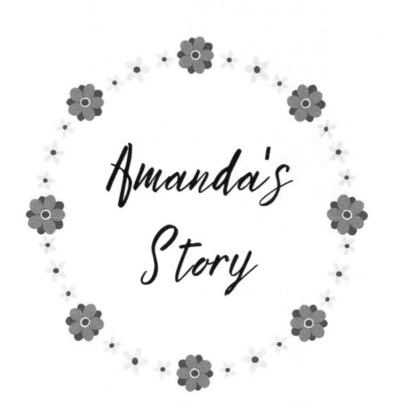

Amanda's Story

My egg donation story – one son and another on the way!

I was diagnosed with POI when I was aged 13 years old after my periods started and stopped at age 11. I was told then that the only way I could have a family was by using donor eggs and IVF – a lot to absorb at just 13.

I spent the rest of my teens in not the best head space, researching all things IVF and egg donation so I have had a pretty in depth understanding from a young age.

My last set of tests from my mid-20s showed one ovary was so small it could hardly be seen and the other was just 0.5cm. I had read many stories of heartache from failed IVF cycles trying to use any remaining eggs and the financial stress, so I drew a line completely under trying with my own eggs in my 20s, even before meeting my now husband, Tom.

I shared my thoughts and feelings on using donor eggs on my YouTube channel and cannot believe how popular it has been. I made a promise to myself when I was 13 that if I did go through IVF with donor eggs that I would share my story and the process as there was no information back then and I wished to help others, I am happy to say it has. It is not easy sharing my story as it's very personal but I know I would have loved that support growing up and in both my IVF cycles.

Fast forward to when I turned 31 and Tom and I embarked on the IVF journey. Using any eggs I may have had left, was never even brought up. I don't believe this was an option anyway from the results of any of my tests. I knew that any child I had as a result of IVF I would love. I couldn't see a reason why I would feel any differently about said child just down to their DNA. I was never really concerned about having a child that looked like me as I know many people that look nothing like their biological parents. I did of course have some concerns like whether I would bond with them in the same way and whether they would accept me once they understood. But these are natural feelings and that's OK!

Egg donor matching

The part I get asked about the most is about the egg matching process. This may vary from clinic to clinic however, you can request as much or as little as you wish – bearing in mind this may have an impact on our quickly you're matched.

You can request skin, hair, eye colours, education, height, build – quite a bit!

For me, I was quite open. I am mixed race (black and white) and was happy for Caucasian, mixed or black donors. My only real request was darker hair and eyes as Tom is quite fair-skinned.

We were matched with a donor that day. I was lucky that a lady had donated her eggs earlier that year and put them in frozen storage as she did not want to wait around to donate. This meant the eggs were ready to go, so the time between our first appointment to transfer was just ten weeks. The donor was my height, my hair colour and my ethnicity – it was meant to be! I was fortunate that our donor left a letter for any child born from her donation which I love to read on a regular basis. Tom even said on paper she sounded like me in personality! We also know from this that she had her own child.

With 'fresh' donor matches, you would have your cycles synced for the donor's egg collection and the sperm will also be collected that same day to fertilise the eggs. You would've had to be on hormone therapy (HRT) to prepare your uterus for transfer which is normally day three or five after transfer. I had no one to sync up with so I just had to increase the size of my uterus ready for transfer. They prefer it to be around 9mm thick and mine was just 2.8mm! Fortunately, my body responded to HRT and it became ready pretty quickly.

We ended up with seven frozen eggs which led to four top grade embryos. We opted for a single embryo transfer (you can have up to two transferred) and they will guide you for your best option from your tests. They gave me 50/50 odds which is quite high in the IVF world and were concerned I would end up with twins.

Well those 50/50 odds produced my now two-year-old, very cheeky, boy Oryn who is my world. As I thought, he is a carbon copy of Tom and many who know our story joke that Tom was cloned! He has slightly darker hair, eyes and skin than Tom but doesn't look remotely mixed-race. This doesn't bother me in the slightest.

Did I bond with him? Do I worry?

My son may look like Tom but his personality is mainly mine! Tom is quiet but Oryn is loud, sings, dances and is sporty (I am a dance, pilates and fitness instructor).

The day he was born he cried, I touched his head and he stared into my eyes and stopped crying. That was it for me. I was his mother. I carried him, grew him, the only person to feel him kick and everything in between. The worries melted away.

I do have low self-esteem, confidence and suffer from anxiety. This is quite understandable when you're diagnosed with something so grown up so young. So yes, toddlers can be mean and if he asks for daddy over me and I am a little low, I can worry it's down to DNA but that is just an insecurity of mine as the next moment he will want me over daddy!

Oryn changed my life. I was so lost; POI took over my life because I let it. I always advise those diagnosed young to enjoy your youth! Do the things you want to do, education, travel whatever it is! It was almost 20 years after my diagnosis that we embarked on IVF – that's a lot of time to be sad when donor eggs have huge success rates.

Worried about the DNA part? Please do not be! Check out my channel or Instagram and see my life with my crazy boy and you can see I couldn't love him any differently! He makes me laugh and smile every single day! I have had strangers say he looks like me too. I personally do not see it but again it doesn't bother me. I know many egg donor mummies and I have never seen a picture of their families and thought 'they look nothing like you'.

I am currently 32 weeks pregnant with my second son from the same batch of embryos as Oryn and we have two remaining in storage. I wish I could go back in time and tell my younger self it would all be ok and that I should live my life a little more.

Will we tell the boys?

Yes. To be honest we have been on TV, in papers and I have my channel, so they would find out anyway but I always wanted to tell them. During fertility treatment, you will see a counsellor that discusses this topic in depth to help you make your own decision. It's a personal choice and I understand both sides. We already have a series of donor egg story books that we read to Oryn and we will keep adapting this as he grows older.

I am proud to say I have received many messages from our story helping people accept donor eggs which has led to several babies being born and they all agree with me that you barely think about the DNA, you're just so in love with that child.

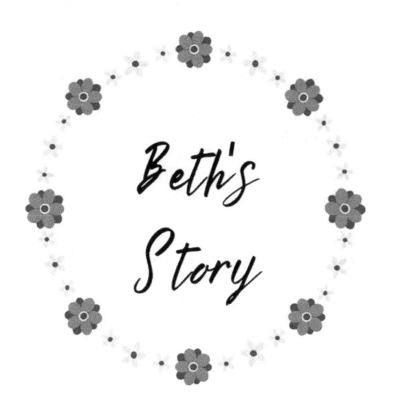

Beth's
Story

When I was diagnosed with POI at 15 years old, the list of symptoms never seemed to end, with the most heart-breaking symptom for me being infertility. Together with one of the most difficult situations of not being able to naturally conceive, was the fact that I started to notice that everyone around me could.

After diagnosis there is no preparation that can be done for what you've to face, the constant feeling of grief over the diagnosis, the want for motherhood or the devastating feeling in the pit of your stomach that each pregnancy announcement brings (or at least this was the case for me) and after so many heart-breaking moments, I had to find a way to get through these announcements.

So, what can be done when faced with a pregnancy announcement of a family member, friend or colleague?

This is a question that I have had to answer many times in the past 10 years and whether it was a friend, family member or colleague, it was always a situation that I struggled to cope with. I found that with every announcement came a mixture of emotions; jealousy, anger and sadness and though this is ok and only normal to feel this way, we must remember not to bottle up these feelings as this could have a negative effect on our mental health.

In the early years of my diagnosis, I struggled to speak to anyone about my feelings, constantly worrying that I would offend those involved or that I would be misunderstood but once I began to open up to friends and family members, I instantly felt a huge weight lifted off my shoulders and though I knew they wouldn't truly understand, they still listened and showed support.

Protecting your mental health is vital and I learnt that self-care is the most important thing for when facing situations like this or any struggles that you could be going through. In my experience, I've found that the top tips for self-care are:

- **Reaching out for support.** Whether it be family, friends, the Daisy Network or medical professions, talking to those around you can provide you with the support you may need. Keeping worries and negative thoughts bottled up can make the struggle worse and can affect your mental health. Always remember, you're never alone in this and there will always be somebody to support you no matter the situation. And I understand that for some (like myself for many years) may struggle to talk to others, so there are other techniques in which to try such as keeping a diary, I kept a diary for six years before I found the Daisy Network and this helped me to express my feelings in my own way.
- **Do what makes YOU happy.** When going through a difficult time, it can be hard to think of doing anything or even getting out of bed! And though it's ok to sometimes take a day or two off, there are ways in which you can overcome this and that is by doing the things that you love. The little moments of happiness like having a relaxing bath, painting or reading, getting out for a little exercise and going for a walk or even snuggling up with your favourite

movie, whatever you enjoy doing, having time for you will improve your mental health.

- **Take your time.** Taking time out for yourself is key when facing tough situations such as pregnancy announcements. You should never feel guilty for taking a step back from the situation and thinking about you. Let yourself rest and care for your mental wellbeing. Mindfulness activities, such as yoga and meditation, are a brilliant way of managing your thoughts and feelings and spending time focusing on you. You should never compare yourself to, or allow yourself to be judged by, others. Only you will know when you're ready and if you don't feel ready to face the friend or family member or attend events such as baby showers then that is ok, do what is best for you.

Facing situations like this with the diagnosis of POI or fertility issues may not be easy and for me, the steps I took for myself made me a stronger woman. It made me strong enough to, after a few weeks, be there for my younger sister as she went through her first pregnancy and though it does not replace the want for motherhood, being an auntie has filled the empty space that infertility left in my heart. If you ever need to chat or would like any support regarding this or POI, please feel free to get in touch with me via the Daisy Network social media pages or by email at bethany@daisynetwork.org.uk

Stay strong through your pain
grow flowers from it
you have helped me
grow flowers from mine so
bloom beautifully
dangerously
loudly
bloom softly
however you need
just bloom

- Rupi Kaur

Daisy Network would like to thank everyone who contributed their stories. Although it takes great bravery and courage, sharing is one of the best ways to not only help heal yourself but heal others too. We know that each of these stories will provide comfort and support by knowing, no matter how you got here, you're not alone on this POI journey.

WHAT WE DO

Our aim as a charity is to provide a support network, both psychological and medical, to those with POI.

As a Daisy Network member, you can find hundreds of others who understand exactly what you're going through. Whether you're newly diagnosed, or 20 years into your diagnosis, our community is a wonderful place to share stories, ask questions and be heard by those who are in the same situation. We provide a private Facebook page for members, regional coordinators who organise local meets-ups and we host a monthly online support group.

We have an incredible medical team who specialise in POI, whether you've a question about your symptoms, medication or fertility, our team provide fortnightly live chats where you can get your questions answered. Our doctors also provide up-to-date knowledge and information within the field of POI and are involved in ongoing research, whilst raising awareness of the condition within the broader medical community.

Find us:

www.daisynetwork.org.uk
Twitter @thedaisynet
Instagram @thedaisynetwork
© 2013-2021 The Daisy Network.
Registered Charity Number 1077930

Author Bios

Amy Bennie is the Chair of Daisy Network. The charity is extremely close to her heart and she has a passion in raising awareness of this relatively unknown condition, and ensuring women with POI receive the medical and psychological support they need throughout their diagnosis. She works as a Counsellor supporting children and adults within the North East.

Kate Maclaran is a Consultant Gynaecologist and subspecialist in Reproductive Medicine at Chelsea Westminster NHS Foundation trust. She is passionate about patient support and raising awareness about Women's Health issues. She leads the unit's fertility support group and is a Trustee of Daisy Network

Catherine o'Keefe Known as Wellness Warrior, is Ireland's first menopause coach and speaker, also running a private practise working with women through menopause. Catherine is founder of the Menopause Success Summit and is an affiliated member of the British Menopause Society.

9 781839 757419